A Manual for Management of
Diabetes Mellitus

A MANUAL FOR MANAGEMENT OF DIABETES MELLITUS
A Hong Kong Chinese Perspective

Revised Edition

Juliana C. N. Chan, Professor
Vincent T. F. Yeung, Consultant
C. C. Chow, Consultant
Gary T. C. Ko, Senior Medical Officer
Clive S. Cockram, Professor of Medicine

Diabetes and Endocrine Centre
Prince of Wales Hospital
and
Department of Medicine and Therapeutics
The Chinese University of Hong Kong

and

Norman N. Chan, Clinical Director

Qualigenics Diabetes Centre
Hong Kong Resort International Limited

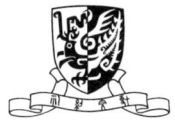

The Chinese University Press

A Manual for Management of Diabetes Mellitus:
A Hong Kong Chinese Perspective (Revised Edition)
By Juliana C. N. Chan, Vincent T. F. Yeung, C. C. Chow,
Gary T. C. Ko, Clive S. Cockram and Norman N. Chan

© **The Chinese University of Hong Kong** 1998, 2005

ISBN 962–996–208–X

First edition 1998
Revised edition 2005

Originally published as *The Prince of Wales Hospital
Manual for Management of Diabetes Mellitus* (Hong Kong:
The Diabetes Centre, Prince of Wales Hospital, 1994)

THE CHINESE UNIVERSITY PRESS
The Chinese University of Hong Kong
Sha Tin, N.T., Hong Kong
Fax: +852 2603 6692
      +852 2603 7355
E-mail: cup@cuhk.edu.hk
Web-site: www.chineseupress.com

Printed in Hong Kong

*This book is dedicated to all diabetic patients
and those involved in their care.
The royalties from the sale of this book
will go to the Prince of Wales Hospital
Diabetes and Endocrine Centre Fund
to improve the quality of care of diabetic patients
and support ongoing research
to advance our understanding of this disease.*

Contents

Foreword by Professor Arthur K. C. Li   xi
Foreword by Dr. Alison M. Reid   xii
Foreword by Professor David Todd   xiii
Foreword by Dr. E. K. Yeoh   xiv
Foreword by Professor Rosie Young   xvi
Preface — Magnitude of the problem of diabetes
   mellitus   xvii
Acknowledgements   xxi
Abbreviations   xxiii

1.   Classification and pathogenesis of diabetes
     mellitus
     1.1   Intermediary metabolism, insulin and
           counter-regulatory hormones   2
     1.2   Classification of diabetes mellitus   2
     1.3   Presentation of diabetes mellitus   3
     1.4   Pathogenesis of diabetes mellitus   4
     1.5   Overlap between Type 1 and Type 2
           diabetes   9
     1.6   Diabetes mellitus in Chinese   10
2.   Diagnosis of diabetes mellitus and impaired
     glucose tolerance
     2.1   Based on venous plasma glucose
           concentration — The ADA and WHO
           criteria   16
     2.2   75 gram oral glucose tolerance test
           (OGTT)   17
     2.3   Diagnosis of impaired glucose
           tolerance   18
3.   Recommended standards of medical care for
     patients with diabetes mellitus
     3.1   Overview   20
     3.2   Initial visit   20
     3.3   Continuing care   23
     3.4   Annual assessment   24
     3.5   Target values   24
     3.6   Hospital admission criteria   26

3.7 Referral for specialist assessment 27

4. Therapeutic patient education
4.1 Health beliefs and affective responses 30
4.2 Knowledge and skills 31
4.3 Rights of patients 31
4.4 Roles of patients 32
4.5 General aspects of treatment 32
4.6 Factors which interfere with glycaemic
control in diabetic patients 32
4.7 Self-monitoring 33
4.8 Insulin administration 35
4.9 Sick day management 36
4.10 Hypoglycaemia 37
4.11 Diabetic complications 41
4.12 Treatment non-compliance 41
4.13 Psycho-sociological problems 42
4.14 Financial aspect 43

5. Dietary management and exercise in diabetes mellitus
5.1 Goals of dietary management 46
5.2 Diet composition 46
5.3 Healthy eating guidelines in diabetes
mellitus 47
5.4 Food choices for diabetic patients 48
5.5 Eating out guidelines 48
5.6 Weight control 49
5.7 Sweeteners (alternatives to sugars) 50
5.8 Exercise 52

6. Oral drug treatment for diabetes mellitus
6.1 Sulphonylureas 56
6.2 Biguanides (metformin) 57
6.3 Thiazolidinediones 58
6.4 Anti-absorptive drugs 59
6.5 Anti-obesity drugs 59
6.6 Oral drug failure (primary or secondary) ... 60
6.7 Combination therapy of insulin and
oral agents 61
6.8 Treatment of Type 2 diabetic patients 63

7. Insulin
7.1 Indications 66
7.2 Actions and duration of insulin 66
7.3 Types of insulin 68

7.4 Regimen 68
7.5 Dosage 70
7.6 Adjustment of dosage 71
7.7 Travelling 74
8. Diabetic complications
8.1 Ophthalmic complications 76
8.2 Diabetic foot 78
8.3 Diabetic neuropathy 82
8.4 Microalbuminuria and renal involvement ... 84
9. Diabetes mellitus and hypertension
9.1 Choices of treatment 90
9.2 Management of hypertension and
    proteinuria in diabetic patients 94
9.3 Use of antihypertensive agents in
    diabetic patients 95
10. Diabetes dyslipidaemia
10.1 Hypercholesterolaemia 98
10.2 Hypertriglyceridaemia 98
10.3 Treatment of hyperlipidaemia 99
10.4 Summary of approaches to diabetic
     patients with dyslipidaemia 101
10.5 Treatment levels and cost-effectiveness
     of lipid lowering drugs 102
11. Peri-operative management
11.1 General principles 106
11.2 Type 2 diabetes — poorly controlled 107
11.3 Type 2 diabetes — well controlled 108
11.4 Type 1 diabetes — poorly controlled 109
11.5 Type 1 diabetes — well controlled 110
12. Diabetic emergencies
12.1 Diabetic ketoacidosis (DKA) 112
12.2 Hyperosmolar non-ketotic coma
     (HNKC) 117
12.3 Lactic acidosis 117
13. Gestational diabetes mellitus
13.1 Definition and prevalence 122
13.2 Screening and diagnosis 122
13.3 Obstetric and perinatal implications 123
13.4 Management 124
14. Prevention of diabetes mellitus
14.1 Primary prevention 130

14.2   Secondary prevention 130
14.3   Tertiary prevention 131
14.4   Multidisciplinary care in diabetes
         mellitus 131

Appendix I.   Body mass index (BMI) chart 133
Appendix II. Carbohydrate exchange list 135
References 139

Foreword

Diabetes mellitus is commonly encountered by doctors of all specialties since the disease can affect different organs and systems. Good knowledge of the condition and its proper management will avoid potentially catastrophic complications and minimize their impacts.

It is therefore both timely and appropriate that a comprehensive set of management guidelines be made available.

The Medical Faculty of the Chinese University of Hong Kong has always striven to be innovative and to provide leadership, excellence and quality in all aspects of clinical care. This set of guidelines fits well with the philosophy of the Faculty and should be of great benefit to the medical staff of hospitals and to general practitioners.

Professor Arthur K. C. Li
Vice-Chancellor
The Chinese University of Hong Kong
1998

Foreword

It is with great pleasure that I contribute to this fine publication. I believe that Prince of Wales Hospital's major strengths are its commitment to teamwork and partnership with the community.

The development of this book is evidence of what is achievable when people from different disciplines work together with a common goal. It also highlights the importance of partnership with patients in the management of diabetes.

Because this book was written with the specific needs of the Hong Kong community in mind, I am confident that it will be an outstanding success. Congratulations to all involved.

Dr. Alison M. Reid
Hospital Chief Executive
Prince of Wales Hospital
1998

Foreword

This is a comprehensive manual on the management of diabetes mellitus which would do a textbook of therapeutics proud. It covers all important and practical aspects of the subject in a language which should be understandable to all health care workers and medical undergraduates. Most of the references are up-to-date. As for useful drugs, a selection is listed so physicians can use those which are most familiar or cost-effective. There is enough pathophysiology to make the text more easily understood. The authors are to be congratulated on producing this manual which should be useful to all those concerned with this subject, and of educational value in undergraduate as well as postgraduate and continuing medical education.

Professor David Todd
President
Hong Kong Academy of Medicine
1998

Foreword

Diabetes mellitus is a serious health problem in Hong Kong affecting an estimated 4.5% of the working population in 1990. More than 50% of the diabetic patients referred to our specialists suffer from complications which give rise to significant mortality and morbidity. These include blindness, end stage renal failure, increased risk of limb amputation and increased susceptibility to infections.

The incidence of diabetes and the related health and social-economic problems are all convincing arguments for enhancing the diagnosis, treatment and care of diabetic patients both in the hospital as well as in the community. However, to achieve such improvements, full participation of patients, medical staff and other health care professionals in an organized programme of education, clinical care and psycho-social support will be required in order to improve the overall health status of diabetic patients.

This book has been written with the objective of providing up-to-date international and local information about the disease to those who are concerned with the care and treatment of diabetes mellitus. The focus is on prevention and self-care, with due emphasis on the importance of co-operation and collaboration between health care professionals, at both the primary care and the hospital level, and the patient.

To complement the advice and information provided in this publication, another book 《積極面對糖尿病》 (Living Positively with Diabetes) has been written specifically for lay people and diabetic patients.

The philosophy of both books is very much in keeping with the Hospital Authority's strategy of developing the role of individuals within the community as Partners and Carers in Health through patient and community education. By working together, we should be able to bring about significant improvements in the treatment and care of diabetic patients in Hong Kong.

Dr. E. K. Yeoh
Chief Executive
Hospital Authority
1998

Foreword

Diabetes mellitus is a worldwide problem. There is growing evidence that the incidence of non-insulin dependent diabetes is rising among the Chinese population in Hong Kong. Changes in demography with more elderly people in the community, a sedentary lifestyle, and unhealthy eating habits are the main factors responsible for this phenomenon. As a chronic illness, diabetes mellitus and its complications not only shorten the life span of an individual but also impair the quality of life and reduce his productivity for many years. Care of diabetic patients also forms an important element of the health budget in Hong Kong.

Good management of diabetes and prevention of diabetic complications require the close co-operation among the health care professionals and full hearted participation of the diabetic patients themselves. This manual for management of diabetes mellitus is comprehensive and easy to read. It gives precise and up-to-date guidance on the management of diabetes and diabetic complications. I would recommend it to all primary care doctors, diabetes nurses and other health care personnel who are interested in diabetes.

Professor Rosie Young
Department of Medicine
The University of Hong Kong
1998

Preface
Magnitude of the problem of diabetes mellitus

Although diabetes mellitus is classified into Type 1, previously known as insulin-dependent diabetes (IDDM) and Type 2, previously known as non-insulin-dependent diabetes (NIDDM), the latter form of diabetes predominates on a global basis and in particular, among non-Caucasians. The prevalence of diabetes has been consistently reported to be between 6–12% among overseas Chinese. In Singapore, the prevalence has doubled from 4% to 8% over a period of 5 years in 1990. In mainland China, the prevalence of diabetes mellitus has increased from <1% in 1990 to 4.5% in 1995. In Hong Kong, the prevalence has been estimated to be 5% in the working population and more than 10% among the elderly in the early 1990s. In 1995, this prevalence of diabetes mellitus was estimated to be 8%, rising from 1.7% in the under 30 years age group to 25% in the elderly. In clinic-based studies, less than 3% of patients have Type 1 diabetes. Even among patients with onset of disease less than the age of 35 years, Type 1 diabetes accounts for less than 10%. Hence, on a local and world-wide basis, Type 2 diabetes represents a major health problem with significant socio-economic impacts.

The mortality rate of diabetic patients is more than double that of the general population. In USA, diabetic patients are 22 times more likely than non-diabetic subjects to be admitted for skin ulcers/gangrene, 15 times more likely for peripheral vascular disease, 6–10 times more for heart disease and cerebrovascular accidents. Hospitalizations for renal disease are accelerated with the risk at 45 years of age or less, being 16 times that of the non-diabetic population. Over one-third of patients on renal replacement therapy have diabetes as a cause of their renal failure. Diabetic patients are 25 times more at risk for blindness. In developed countries, including Hong Kong, diabetes is the leading cause of blindness in adults of working age. Hospitalizations for eye disease are also more common in diabetic patients 65 years of age or less.

In Hong Kong, over 50% of diabetic patients attending hospital clinics have coexisting hypertension, dyslipidaemia and/or increased albuminuria. Cardiovascular and cerebro-vascular diseases are the second and third leading causes of death in Hong Kong. Among patients admitted with cerebrovascular accident, between 15% and 30% of patients have history of diabetes or are diagnosed as a result of the stroke. Over 25% of patients admitted with acute myocardial infarction have diabetes as a risk factor. Of the 100 amputations performed in a regional hospital each year, over 50% are due to diabetes. Between 15% and 30% of patients on long-term renal replacement therapy have diabetes as their causes of renal failure. Over 200 diabetic patients become blind every year.

The close associations between hypertension, dyslipidaemia and Type 2 diabetes are now well documented. These risk factors contribute independently to the increased mortality and morbidity of diabetic patients. **GENETIC FACTORS**, **AGEING** and environmental determinants are important in the pathogenesis of these diseases. The prevalence of diabetes varies from less than 1% in some rural areas in mainland China to as high as 16% amongst Chinese living in Mauritius. To date, the identifiable predictive factors for diabetes include **OBESITY** (particularly **central obesity** with increased abdominal fat), **PHYSICAL INACTIVITY** and other yet to be identified aspects of **URBANIZATION** (e.g. diet, stress). Correction of some of these environmental factors, i.e. **modification of lifestyle**, is useful in the primary prevention of these diseases and should be emphasized in patients with these conditions. The results of the Diabetes Control and Complication Trial (DCCT) have shown that good glycaemic control is associated with a 60% reduction in the development and progression of microangiopathic complications in Type 1 diabetes. Similar results have also been reported in insulin-treated Type 2 diabetic patients. In established cases of diabetes, the aims of treatment include **relief of symptoms, reduction of long-term complications, improvement of quality of life and well-being and treatment of associated conditions**.

The essence of management of diabetes mellitus lies primarily in prevention. This relies on adequate co-operation between health care providers and patients. Emphasis on patient SELF-CARE through effective

therapeutic patient education programmes and continuing update of the health care providers are fundamental.

This manual, which combines the latest international and local guidelines for the management of diabetes and consists of data based on local research, was prepared by a team of doctors at the Diabetes and Endocrine Centre of the Prince of Wales Hospital, and Department of Medicine and Therapeutics, The Chinese University of Hong Kong. It aims to provide a quick reference to all health care personnel involved in the management of diabetes mellitus with emphasis upon Type 2 diabetes.

The ideal management of diabetes mellitus involves a **MULTI-DISCIPLINARY** approach. The patient is the core of the team, supplemented by the primary health care providers for the day to day management of the disease. The Diabetes and Endocrine Centre provides comprehensive diabetic complication screening and education programmes and specialized treatments as required. With the support of the Department of Health (N.T. East) of the Hong Kong Government, the PWH Diabetes and Endocrine Centre has adopted this shared care approach. This manual represents one of the education materials prepared in conjunction with the implementation of this shared care programme in order to provide updated information in the management of this serious but highly preventable disease. We hope this will eventually lead to a significant improvement in diabetes care within our community.

Acknowledgements

We are indebted to formerly Professor Patrick Ho, Eye Unit; Dr. S. F. Lui, Consultant, Renal Unit and Chief of Service, Medical Unit; Professor Brian Tomlinson, Division of Clinical Pharmacology, Department of Medicine and Therapeutics, The Chinese University of Hong Kong, for their expert and invaluable comments.

We also thank Ms. Rebecca Wong, Ms. Eva Kan and Ms. Kit Man Lo, Diabetes Nurse Specialists, and Ms. Rita Lo and Ms. Lulu Lam, our dietitians at the Prince of Wales Hospital for their contributions. Specific thanks are extended to Dr. C. Y. Li, our Consultant Obstetrician, for contributing the chapter on gestational diabetes mellitus, and to Ms. Janet Lok, Manager of the Dietetic Department, Prince of Wales Hospital, for rewriting the chapter on dietary management and exercise.

We are most grateful to the following pharmaceutical companies for their contributions which make the establishment of the Prince of Wales Hospital Diabetes and Endocrine Centre a possibility. These companies are listed as follows:

Armedic-Servier Far East Ltd.
Bayer Diagnostics China Co. Ltd.
Boehringer Mannheim China Ltd.
Bristol-Myers Squibb (Hong Kong) Ltd.
Eisai (Hong Kong) Co. Ltd.
Eli Lilly Asia Inc. (Hong Kong Branch)
Hoechst China Ltd.
Johnson & Johnson Medical Hong Kong
Novo Nordisk, Swire Loxley Ltd.
Parke-Davis, Warner-Lambert (Hong Kong) Ltd.
Pharmacia, Farmitalia Carlo Erba (Hong Kong) Ltd.

Our deepest thanks are also extended to Dr. K. H. Mak, the Community Physician of the Department of Health (N.T. East) and the Shatin District Board. Without their support, this shared care programme would not have been a reality.

Abbreviations

4S	Scandinavian Simvastatin Survival Study
ACE	angiotensin converting enzyme
ACEI	angiotensin converting enzyme inhibitor
ACR	albumin:creatinine ratio
ADA	American Diabetes Association
AER	albumin excretion rate
AII	angiotensin II
ARB	angiotensin II receptor blocker
BG	blood glucose
BMI	body mass index
BP	blood pressure
CCB	calcium channel blocking agents
CHD	coronary heart disease
CPK	creatine phosphate kinase
CVP	central venous pressure
CVSRF	cardiovascular risk factor
CXR	chest radiograph
DCCT	Diabetes Control and Complication Trial
DKA	diabetic ketoacidosis
DKI	dextrose/potassium/insulin
DM	diabetes mellitus
DNA	deoxyribonucleic acid
ECG	electrocardiogram
FFA	free fatty acid
FPG	fasting plasma glucose
GAD	glutamic acid decarboxylase
GDM	gestational diabetes mellitus
GH	growth hormone
HbA_{1c}	glycated haemoglobin
HDL-C	high density lipoprotein cholesterol
HM	human
HMG-CoA	hydroxymethylglutaryl-coenzyme A
HNF	hepatic nuclear factor
HNKC	hyperosmolar non-ketotic coma
IDL-C	intermediate density lipoprotein cholesterol
IFG	impaired fasting glucose
IGT	impaired glucose tolerance

IV	intravenous
IZS	zinc suspension insulin
LADA	late onset autoimmune diabetes in adults
LDL-C	low density lipoprotein cholesterol
LVH	left ventricular hypertrophy
MC	monocomponent
MODY	maturity onset diabetes of the young
NDDG	National Diabetes Data Group
NFG	normal fasting glucose
NPH	neutral protamine hagedorn
NS	normal saline
OCP	oral contraceptive pills
OGTT	oral glucose tolerance test
PR	pulse rate
RAS	renin angiotensin system
RFT	renal function test
SBGM	self blood glucose monitoring
SIADH	syndrome of inappropriate anti-diuretic hormone
SNS	sympathetic nervous system
TB	tuberculosis
TC	total cholesterol
TG	triglyceride
TZD	thiazolidinediones
UAE	urinary albumin excretion
VLDL-C	very low density lipoprotein cholesterol
VSMC	vascular smooth muscle cell
WHO	World Health Organization
WHR	waist-to-hip ratio

Chapter **1**

Classification and pathogenesis of diabetes mellitus

1.   Classification and pathogenesis

1.1 Intermediary metabolism, insulin and counter-regulatory hormones

- diabetes is a complex and heterogeneous disease, characterized by chronic hyperglycaemia
- it is a disorder of energy metabolism due to either a deficiency of insulin action (qualitative or quantitative) or enhanced activity of the counter-regulatory hormones or both
- inability to use glucose effectively for energy production or storage results in chronic hyperglycaemia, which is translated to vascular abnormalities and tissue damages

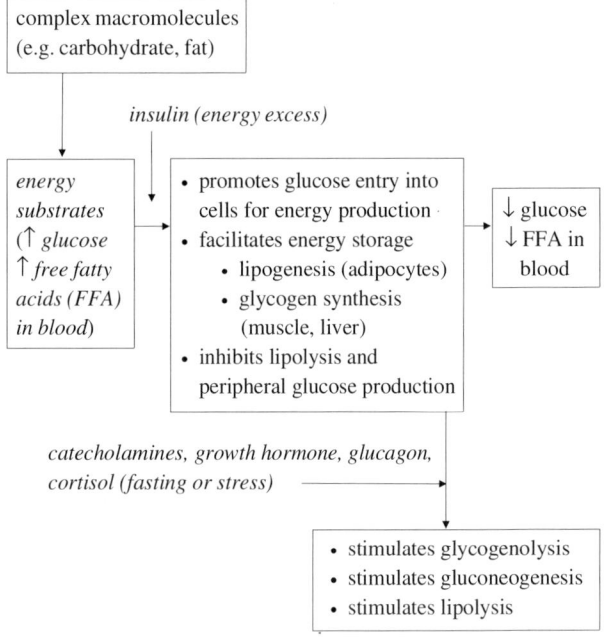

Fig. 1.1   Intermediary metabolism, insulin and counter-regulatory hormones

1.2 Classification of diabetes mellitus

- the pathogenesis of diabetes mellitus has both environmental and genetic determinants as reflected by the

marked variations in prevalence in different countries and within ethnic groups living in different areas
- increasing number of subgroups of diabetes mellitus are being identified

Table 1.1 The classification of diabetes mellitus by the American Diabetes Association (ADA) (1997)

1 Type 1 diabetes (β cell destruction, usually leading to absolute insulin deficiency)
- immune mediated
- idiopathic
2 Type 2 diabetes (may range from predominantly insulin resistance with relative insulin deficiency to a predominantly secretory defect with insulin resistance)
3 Other specific types
- genetic defects of b cell function
  - chromosome 12, HNF 1α (formerly MODY 3)
  - chromosome 7, glucokinase (formerly MODY 2)
  - chromosome 20, HNF 4α (formerly MODY 1)
  - mitochrondrial DNA
- genetic defects in insulin action
- diseases of exocrine pancreas
- endocrinopathies (e.g. Cushing's syndrome, acromegaly, phaeochromocytoma,, glucagonoma)
- drug or chemical induced
- infections
- uncommon forms of immune mediated diabetes
- other genetic syndromes sometimes associated with diabetes
- gestational diabetes mellitus

MODY = maturity onset diabetes of the young
HNF = hepatic nuclear factor

1.3 Presentation of diabetes mellitus

1.3.1 Type 1 diabetes in Caucasians

- autoimmune Type 1 diabetes, characterized by absolute insulin deficiency, is the predominant form of diabetes mellitus in Caucasian patients with young onset of disease (<35 years)
- ketosis-prone
- acute symptoms

- non-obese
- complications unlikely within the first 5 years of diagnosis

1.3.2   Type 2 diabetes

- over 95% of diabetic patients in the world have Type 2 diabetes
- predominant form of diabetes among non-Caucasians, young and old
- non-ketosis prone
- obese or non-obese
- frequently missed
- often complicated at presentation
- often part of a multifaceted "Metabolic Syndrome" in the majority of patients (see 1.4.5)

Note:

- small amount of ketones in urine (<3+) in Type 2 diabetic patients may be due to relatively insufficient insulin action to inhibit lipolysis and ketone body formation
- insufficient carbohydrate intake resulting in fat being used as an alternate fuel substrate can also lead to ketonuria

1.4 Pathogenesis of diabetes mellitus

1.4.1   Type 1 diabetes

- **autoimmunity** is the main cause of Type 1 diabetes in Caucasians
  - lymphocytic infiltration of pancreatic β cell with cellular destruction and severe insulin deficiency
  - presence of autoantibodies to various islet cell autoantigens
  - association with other autoimmune diseases, e.g. autoimmune thyroiditis, premature ovarian failure
- several triggers for the immunological events have been implicated but none are proven, e.g. viruses, chemical toxins, cow's milk antigens
- **antibodies to glutamic acid decarboxylase** (GAD):
  - GAD has been identified as the 64K autoantigen in the pancreatic islets cells

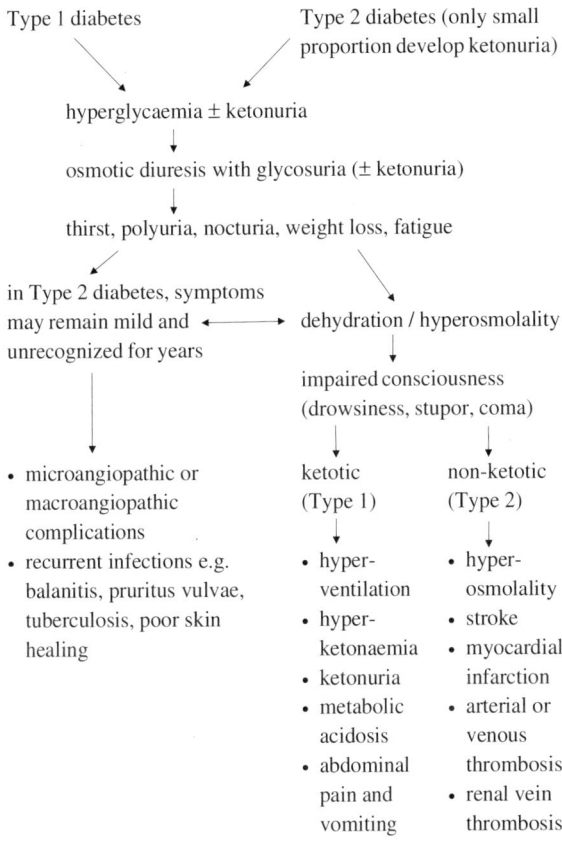

Fig. 1.2   **Classical presenting features of Type 1 and Type 2 diabetes**

- predict the onset of Type 1 diabetes in Caucasians
- detectable in >70% of newly diagnosed Caucasian Type 1 diabetic patients and >50% of patients with long duration of disease (>5 years)
- marked variations in the prevalence of antibodies to GAD among different ethnic groups
- low prevalence of anti-GAD in non-Caucasian Type 1 diabetic patients
- prevalence of anti-GAD in Hong Kong Chinese:
  - 12% in young subjects (age of onset <35 years)
  - 20% in young patients with insulin deficiency

– 30% in young patients with both insulin deficiency and acute presentation

1.4.2 Type 2 diabetes

- marked heterogeneity characterized by **insulin resistance** and **relative insulin deficiency**, both of which have genetic and environmental determinants
- although insulin resistance is a strong predictor for Type 2 diabetes, insulin deficiency plays a critical role in the development of overt diabetes
- subtle defects in insulin secretion are demonstrable in patients with mild glucose intolerance as well as in normoglycaemic relatives of diabetic subjects
- the degree of insulin deficiency required for diabetes to manifest is related to the degree of underlying insulin resistance

1.4.3 Insulin deficiency

- pre-synthesized insulin is stored in the pancreatic islet

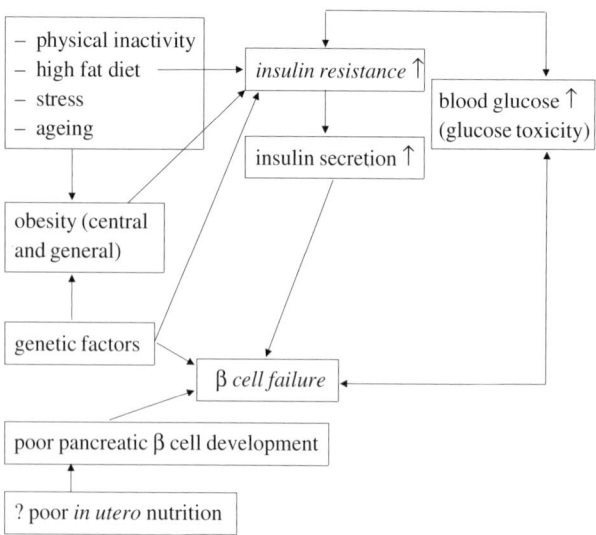

Fig. 1.3 Pathogenesis of Type 2 diabetes

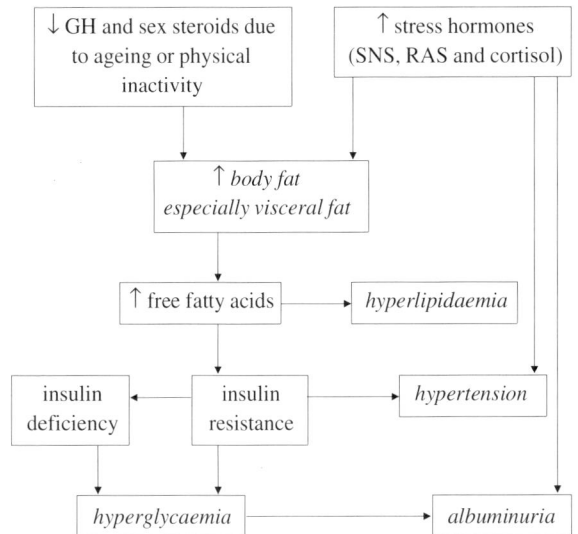

SNS = sympathetic nervous system
RAS = renin angiotensin system
GH = growth hormone

Fig. 1.4   Visceral Fat Syndrome (Metabolic Syndrome)

• increased free fatty acid (FFA) formation may induce insulin resistance by increasing gluconeogenesis and reducing glucose uptake in the muscles, the interactions between these neurohormonal systems may give rise to metabolic and vascular manifestations

1.5 Overlap between Type 1 and Type 2 diabetes

• there is considerable overlap between the clinical manifestations of Type 1 and Type 2 diabetes making differentiation on pure clinical grounds sometimes difficult

1.5.1   Late onset autoimmune diabetes in adults (LADA)

• slow onset and non-ketotic presentation
• insulin deficient with detectable antibodies to GAD
• rapid oral drug failure requiring continuous insulin treatment shortly after diagnosis

1.5.2 Flatbush diabetes (Type 1½ diabetes)

- reported in Afro-Americans and also seen in Chinese, presenting with ketoacidosis but subsequently revert to a clinical course resembling Type 2 diabetes
- non-insulin deficient as a predominant feature but insulin resistant
- acute presentation due to insulin resistance aggravated by relative insulin deficiency and glucose toxicity
- often obese
- negative for antibodies to GAD

1.5.3 Maturity onset diabetes of the young (MODY)

- due to genetic defects of β-cell functions
- diabetes diagnosed before the age of 25
- treatable without insulin for more than 5 years
- negative for antibodies to islet cells or GAD
- different subgroups have been described in various population with mutations in glucokinase, HNF 1α and HNF 4α (see Table 1.1)

1.5.4 Subgroups of diabetes due to genetic defects

- some examples:
  - insulin mutation → impaired insulin secretion
  - insulin receptor mutation → insulin resistance
  - insulin receptor substrate-1 mutation → insulin resistance
  - mitochondrial DNA mutation → insulin deficiency, high tone deafness, maternal history of diabetes

1.6 Diabetes mellitus in Chinese

- using the World Health Organization (WHO) criteria, the prevalence ranges from less than 1% in some rural areas in mainland China to over 16% in some overseas Chinese (Fig. 1.5)
- the prevalence of diabetes mellitus in Hong Kong Chinese has increased from 4.5% in 1990 to 7.9% in 1995 (Figs. 1.6, 1.7)
- main predictive factors for diabetes mellitus include:
  - increased age

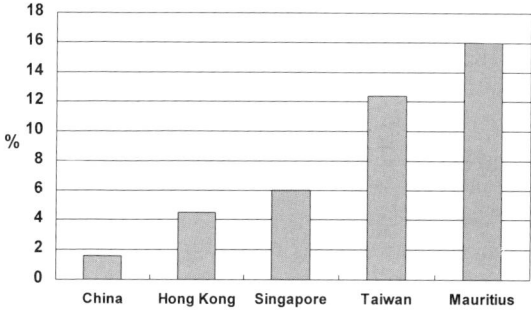

Fig. 1.5   Diabetes mellitus in Chinese populations

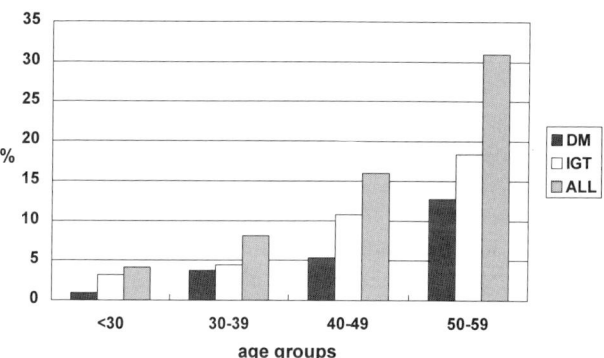

Fig. 1.6   Prevalence of glucose intolerance in Hong Kong Chinese, 1990

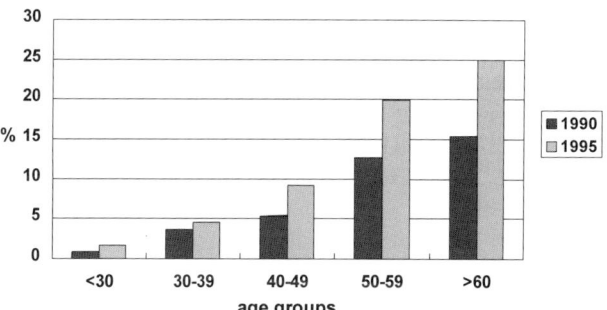

Fig. 1.7   Prevalence of diabetes mellitus in Hong Kong Chinese, 1990 and 1995

- obesity (body mass index (BMI) and waist-to-hip ratio (WHR))
- family history
- high personal income especially in subjects with low education level
- physical inactivity
- pattern of diabetes in Hong Kong Chinese
  - mean age only 50 years with over 20 years of follow up
  - 3% have Type 1 presentation (ketosis prone or continuous insulin treatment within 1 year of diagnosis)
    - poor correlation with pancreatic beta cell function
  - Type 2 patients
    - 25% require insulin treatment
    - 30% have positive family history
    - 50% have coexisting hypertension, dyslipidaemia and increased albuminuria
  - leading causes of death
    - 3% annual mortality rate mainly due to cardiovascular events and renal failure
    - HbA_{1c} and albuminuria are independent predictors for death
- Hong Kong Chinese patients with young onset of disease
  - 20% of clinic population
  - 10% have Type 1 presentation
  - 10% have antibodies to islet cell antigen, e.g. GAD
  - poor correlation between pancreatic beta cell function and presenting features
  - 50% require insulin treatment
  - 50% are insulin deficient
  - 50% have positive family history
  - 10% have genetic mutations (glucokinase, hepatic nuclear factor (HNF), amylin, mitochondrial DNA) known to cause insulin secretory failure
- health care used by Hong Kong Chinese diabetic patients
  - 40% of admissions to medical wards involve diabetes mellitus
  - 30% of patients with renal failure, stroke, heart failure, myocardial infarction, have diabetes as a major contributory factor
  - 30% of patients have retinopathy at the time of referral
  - 200 new cases of blindness due to diabetes per year

- 50% of admissions due to adverse drug reactions are related to drug-induced hypoglycaemia
  - renal failure and increased age are major associated factors
- 60% of patients attending hospital clinics have cardio-vascular diseases and/or risk factors
- 30% of prescriptions issued contain anti-diabetic drugs

Chapter **2**

Diagnosis of diabetes mellitus and impaired glucose tolerance

2. Diagnosis of diabetes mellitus

- in view of the chronic nature of the disease and its potential complications, it is important to establish an early diagnosis of diabetes mellitus especially in high risk individuals
- abnormal blood glucose levels during stresses (illnesses or medications which affect glucose tolerance) and in the absence of diabetic complications or previous symptoms suggestive of diabetes are usually interpreted as "**stress hyperglycaemia**," which should be re-assessed after the acute event is over, preferably after 6 weeks or more.

2.1 Based on venous plasma glucose concentration — The ADA and WHO criteria

patients at risk:
- elderly, obese, positive family history, hypertension, hyperlipidaemia, history of GDM or stress-induced hyperglycaemia

symptoms of diabetes:
- weight loss, thirst, polyuria, lethargy, balanitis, pruritus vulvae, recurrent infection

random plasma glucose ⟶ ≥11.1 mmol/l

7–11 mmol/l

fasting plasma glucose ⟶ ≥7.0 mmol/l

<6.0 mmol/l   6.1–7.0 mmol/l

impaired fasting glucose (IFG)
(may consider to perform 75 g OGTT to diagnosis IGT)

normal fasting glucose (NFG)
- diabetes unlikely in asymptomatic or low risk subjects

2-hr plasma glucose ≥11.1 mmol/l ⟶

diabetes mellitus
- in asymptomatic subjects, 2 abnormal values are required

impaired glucose tolerance, IGT (WHO criteria)
- fasting plasma glucose <7.0 mmol/l
- 2-hr plasma glucose 7.8–11.1 mmol/l

- assess other cardiovascular risk factors (BP, lipid, weight, smoking)
- emphasize healthy lifestyle
- test fasting plasma glucose and other risk factors 1–2 yearly

Note:

- conversion factor: mmol/l = mg/dl ÷ 18
- plasma glucose ≈ whole blood glucose × 1.12
- venous plasma glucose concentration is recommended for diagnostic purpose
- diagnosis by capillary blood glucose using finger prick test is not recommended
- urinalysis is not diagnostic
- the reproducibility of 75 gram OGTT is only 50% and
- the ADA recommendation omits the use of 75 gram OGTT and bases the diagnosis only on fasting plasma glucose
- 11.1 mmol/l is the threshold value of plasma glucose for development of retinopathy
- the definition of diagnostic fasting plasma glucose (FPG) is more arbitrary and most studies have shown that the FPG corresponding to a 2-hr value of 11.1 mmol/l is less than 7.0 mmol/l
- in Hong Kong Chinese, this value lies somewhere between 5.6 and 6.0 mmol/l
- reducing the diagnostic FPG value from 7.8 mmol/l to 7.0 mmol/l increases the sensitivity of this test to diagnose diabetes from 20% to 40%, hence in high risk subjects, a 75 g OGTT may still need to be performed to diagnose subjects with 2-hr post glucose loading plasma glucose ≥11.1 mmol/l

2.2 75 gram oral glucose tolerance test (OGTT)

- not recommended as a routine test due to its labour intensity, high cost and poor reproducibility (~50%)
- principally used when blood glucose levels are equivocal, during pregnancy or in epidemiological surveys
- should be administered in the morning after at least 3 days of unrestricted diet (150 g of carbohydrate daily), usual physical activity and preceded by an overnight fast of 10–16 hours, during which time water may be drunk
- no smoking is permitted during the test or overnight prior to the test
- no major operation or illness 6 weeks before test

- document medications
- use 75 g anhydrous glucose
- the WHO value of fasting plasma glucose for diagnosing diabetes is 7.0 mmol/l

2.3 Diagnosis of impaired glucose tolerance

- IGT can only be diagnosed by OGTT
- diagnosis made when FPG is < 7.0 mmol/l and 2-hour glucose is between 7.8 and 11.1 mmol/l

Chapter **3**

Recommended standards of medical care for patients with diabetes mellitus

3. Recommended standards of medical care for patients with diabetes mellitus

3.1 Overview

- comprehensive assessment
    - lifestyle factors, family history
    - complications and risk factors
    - glycaemic control (HbA_{1c})
- therapeutic patient education
    - knowledge, attitude, behaviour modification
    - health beliefs
    - skills
    - patient empowerment and self-care
- regular follow up and periodic assessment

3.2 Initial visit

3.2.1 History taking

- symptoms of hyperglycaemia and diabetic complications
- laboratory tests for the diagnosis of diabetes
- history of ketoacidosis
- dietary habits, weight and exercise history
- previous treatment programmes and diabetes education
- current medications (antidiabetic drugs, steroids, diuretics, antihypertensive drugs, oral contraceptives)
- self-monitoring (urine or blood)
- plan for pregnancy
- identify other risk factors:
    - smoking
    - hypertension
    - hyperlipidaemia
    - family history (diabetes, hypertension, kidney and cardiovascular diseases)
    - gestational diabetes or large babies (>4.5 kg)
- other significant past medical history including tuberculosis

3.2.2 Complete physical examination with particular emphasis on:

- general state: hydration, xanthelesma, tendon and eruptive xanthomata, carotid bruit

- body weight and height
- ideal body weight as estimated by:
  body mass index (**BMI** = kg ÷ m ÷ m = kg/m^2 (see Appendix I for BMI chart)
- obesity as defined by the National Diabetes Data Group (NDDG): >27 kg/m^2 in male, >25 kg/m^2 in female
- mean BMI among Hong Kong Chinese <65 years old is between 23–24 kg/m^2?
- central adiposity (an index of insulin resistance) by measuring the waist-to-hip ratio (**WHR**). The waist circumference is the minimum circumference between the umbilicus and xiphoid process, the hip circumference is the maximum circumference around the buttock and symphysis pubis
- mean WHR among Chinese <65 years old is between 0.8–0.9
- blood pressure (ideal blood pressure: ≤130/80 mmHg; normotension: ≤140/90 mmHg) and examine for left ventricular hypertrophy or cardiomegaly
- visual acuity and ophthalmoscopic examination, if possible with dilatation unless contraindicated (e.g. history of glaucoma)
- abdomen (hepatomegaly often due to fatty changes)
- foot evaluation especially deformities, skin condition, fungal infection, foot pulses and neurological examination (vibration sense, touch, ankle jerks) (see 8.2)
- possible secondary causes for diabetes (thyrotoxicosis, acromegaly, Cushing's syndrome, phaeochromocytoma) especially in young diabetic patients with atypical presentations

3.2.3 Laboratory evaluation

- fasting plasma glucose concentration
- glycated haemoglobin (HbA$_{1c}$)
- fasting serum lipid profile
  - total cholesterol (TC), triglyceride (TG) and high density lipoprotein cholesterol (HDL-C) especially if treatment with lipid lowering agent is considered
  - calculate low density lipoprotein cholesterol (LDL-C) using the Friedewald's equation:

$$TC = HDL\text{-}C + LDL\text{-}C + (TG \div 2.2) \text{ if } TG < 4.5 \text{ (all values measured in mmol/l)}$$

- dipstix examination of urine for ketones, glucose and protein (detection for microalbuminuria preferred if available, also see 8.4.3)
- perform urine culture and microscopy if dipstix examination is abnormal or patient is symptomatic
- 24-hr urinary protein excretion if albustix is positive in sterile samples
- baseline renal and liver function tests
- ECG if symptomatic or hypertensive
- CXR (if not done within last 3 years) or in the presence of symptoms

3.2.4 Management plan

- set a realistic and mutually agreed goal for each patient:
  - relieve symptoms
  - prevent acute and chronic complications
  - reduce the rate of progression of complications
  - improve quality of life
- avoid over treatment in the elderly and patients with reduced life span in whom symptomatic relief and avoidance of acute metabolic decompensation are the main treatment goals
- explain nature of disease, rationale for treatment and emphasize compliance
- emphasize **self-care** through patient and family education (dietitians, diabetes nurses, podiatrists if available)
- teach self-monitoring techniques (blood/urine) and appropriate responses for the results
- nutritional recommendations and exercise programme (simple advice such as "eat less" and "walk more" can be repeatedly emphasized)
- referral to a podiatrist if foot is at risk (absent pulses, neuropathy, deformities, history of lower extremity amputation)
- discuss contraception and review of diabetes care **before** and during pregnancy
- see 3.7 for referral for specialist assessment

3.3 Continuing care

3.3.1 Visit frequency

a) insulin-treated patients:
*   frequent contact (e.g. by phone) at the clinic or a diabetes day centre as often as daily may be required in patients starting insulin or having a major change in their insulin regimen until:
    – blood glucose control is adequate
    – risk of hypoglycaemia is low
    – patient is competent to carry out treatment plan
*   at least 3–4 monthly follow up if stable

b)   non-insulin treated patients:
*   may be weekly contact (e.g. by phone) until control is stable
*   at least 6 monthly if stable
*   not more than 1 month if there have been major changes in treatment

3.3.2 At each visit

*   evaluate the treatment goals
*   review new problems and medical history
*   assess frequency, causes and severity of hypo- and hyper-glycaemic episodes
*   assess and discuss the results of self-monitoring with patients
*   review adjustment of the therapeutic regimen by patients
*   check treatment compliance
*   physical examination
    – body weight
    – blood pressure
    – appropriate examination as indicated by medical history
*   laboratory evaluation
    – plasma glucose (fasting or post-prandial) at least 3 monthly
    – HbA_{1c} at least 6 monthly (preferably 3 monthly) for insulin-treated patients and in non-insulin treated patients with poor glycaemic control

3.4 Annual assessment

- complete physical examination including:
  - ophthalmoscopy through dilated pupils and visual acuity (corrected with glasses or pinhole if necessary)
  - foot examination including skin, deformities, pulses, sensation (vibration, touch) and reflexes
  - blood pressure (lying and standing)
- laboratory tests:
  - HbA$_{1c}$
  - fasting plasma lipid (TC, TG, HDL-C) and calculate LDL-C
  - urine for protein and preferably albumin excretion (after exclusion of infection) — see 8.4.3 for methods of collection
  - renal function test (plasma Na$^+$, K$^+$, urea and creatinine)
  - liver function test especially if patient is treated with metformin

3.5 Target values

3.5.1 Targets for body weight, blood pressure and glycaemic control

	Optimal*	Borderline	Undesirable
plasma glucose (mmol/l)			
– fasting	4–7	7–10	>10
– random	4–8	8–12	>12
HbA$_{1c}$** (%)	<7	7–8.5	>8.5
BMI (kg/m^2) (under 65 years old)	19–24	24–25	>25
WHR (under 65 years old)	<0.9	0.9–1.0	>1.0
systolic BP*** (mmHg)	<130	135–140	>140
diastolic BP*** (mmHg)	<80	85–95	>95

* • This is the ideal treatment goal. Individualization of treatment plan is important.
   • Balance the risk of hypoglycaemia due to intensive treatment against its benefits especially in elderly patients and those with reduced life span or poor quality of life.

- For young patients, optimal control should be the primary aim due to long duration of disease.
- The risk of microangiopathic complications increases sharply once HbA$_{1c}$ exceeds 8.5%.

** The values of HbA$_{1c}$ may vary between laboratories. **Values quoted are results obtained from ion exchange chromatography. For other assays, values which are ≤1.1 and ≥1.4 times the upper limit of normal range may be used as the optimal and undesirable values, respectively.**

*** Avoid precipitous fall in blood pressure (BP) in the elderly and in those suffering from known cerebrovascular atherosclerosis. Optimal BP control may not be always possible but one should always aim to achieve the lowest tolerable BP.

3.5.2 Targets for control of fasting serum lipid levels

	Optimal*	Borderline	Undesirable
TC	<5.2	5.2–6.1	≥6.2
HDL-C	>1.1	0.9–1.1	0.9
LDL-C	<2.6	2.6–3.2	≥3.2
TG	<1.7	1.7–2.3	≥2.4

- interactions between lipid levels and other cardiovascular risk factors are more important than absolute values
- in patients with a history of cardiovascular diseases (e.g. stroke, myocardial ischaemia, peripheral vascular disease, leg amputation)
- aim at   HDL-C > 0.9 (preferably ≥1.2) mmol/l
               LDL-C ≤ 2.6 mmol/l
               TG ≤ 1.7 mmol/l
- if HDL-C ≤0.9 mmol/l or hypertensive or smoker
  aim at   LDL-C <3.4 mmol/l
  TG <2.3 mmol/l
- if LDL-C/HDL-C >5 mmol/l aim at TG <2.3 mmol/l
- HDL-C ≥1.4 mmol/l and a pre-menopausal state are protective against coronary heart disease

3.5.3   Clinical protocol

At initial visit

Complete examination
- BMI, WHR
- blood pressure
- foot inspection
- fundoscopy
- visual acuity
- CXR/ECG (as indicated)

Biochemical tests
- plasma glucose
- HbA$_{1c}$
- fasting serum lipid profile
- renal function
- urine glucose, protein, ketones, microscopy
- microalbuminuria

Start teaching programme
- lifestyle modification including dietary advice
- teach self-monitoring

At second visit

Continue teaching programme
- body weight
- blood pressure
- plasma glucose

Every 3 months

Continue teaching programme
- body weight
- blood pressure
- plasma glucose

Every 6 months
- HbA$_{1c}$
- fasting serum lipid profile (if $\uparrow$)
- urine protein (if $\uparrow$)
- foot inspection (if at risk)

Annually
- complete examination and biochemical tests
- check self-monitoring technique
- re-evaluate therapy and treatment goals
- referral to specialist care for assessment if progress is unsatisfactory

3.6 Hospital admission criteria

- severe acute metabolic complications of diabetes (e.g. frequent hypo- or hyperglycaemic episodes)
- newly diagnosed diabetes in children and adolescents
- poor metabolic control requiring close monitoring to define cause and modify therapy

- severe chronic complications requiring intensive treatment
- co-existing conditions, e.g. severe infection that significantly affects diabetic control and requires treatment modification
- uncontrolled or newly diagnosed insulin-requiring diabetes during pregnancy
- commencement of intensive insulin treatment regimes (e.g. multiple injections or continuous subcutaneous insulin infusion) if unsuccessful on an outpatient basis

3.7 Referral for specialist assessment

- ketotic, poor general condition at presentation
- failure to achieve satisfactory control of glycaemia as evidenced by, e.g. persistent weight loss, ketonuria, fasting plasma glucose >15 mmol/l
- failure to achieve acceptable control of associated conditions, e.g. hypertension and hyperlipidaemia (see 3.5 for target values)
- starting insulin treatment
- foot problems, e.g. resistant skin infection, non-healing ulcers, vascular complications (e.g. intermittent claudication, absent foot pulses)
- ophthalmic complications, e.g. cataract with visual impairment, retinopathy, visual impairment not corrected by pinhole
- persistent proteinuria and rising plasma creatinine concentration
- cardiovascular complications such as ischaemic heart disease, heart failure
- neuropathy especially if symptomatic

Chapter 4

Therapeutic patient education

4. Therapeutic patient education

- effective diabetes education improves glycaemic control and is therapeutic
- **without appropriate diabetes education, adequate glycaemic control can rarely be achieved**
- although in-depth diabetes education can be provided by health care providers such as diabetes nurses, dietitians and podiatrists, doctors should take a leading role and outline the principles of management to patients in simple terms
- aim to provide encouragement and ongoing education to reinforce and update skills and knowledge
- positive **attitudes** as well as **knowledge** are both important for **behaviour modification**
- use educational aids such as information kits, slide-tapes, flip charts and videotapes for large classes and individualized education sessions
- involve the family members particularly with elderly patients
- **patient empowerment: make the patient a member of the management team and emphasize the importance of self-care**

4.1 Health beliefs and affective responses

- diabetes mellitus is a chronic disease, which is frequently asymptomatic and can be associated with major complications
- patients' active participation is required if treatment goal is to be achieved
- patients should have correct health beliefs
  - they are at risk of diabetic complications
  - these complications constitute a serious threat to their health
  - these complications can be kept under control or cured
  - the psychological, social and financial costs of the treatment are less than the benefits of the treatment
- the affective responses of the patients should be appreciated by the health care providers
  - patients' psychology in coping with the disease
    - denial, revolt, bargaining, depression, acceptance

- help patients to develop positive attitude and value clarification
- provide emotional support to patients and carers
- help patients to develop responsibility for self-care (rights and roles of a diabetic patient)
- to empower patients to gain internal control

4.2 Knowledge and skills

- knowledge
  - nature, causes, symptoms and signs of diabetes
  - treatment principles: meal planning, exercise and drugs
  - acute complications: causes and management of hypo- and hyperglycaemia
  - chronic complications: aetiology, prevention and treatment
  - long-term goals: optimal body weight, BP, lipid and glycaemic control
  - special issues: foot care, sick day management and travelling
  - smoking and alcohol
  - impotence, contraception and planned pregnancy
  - gestational diabetes
- skills
  - insulin injection: insulin syringe, insulin pen, storage of insulin, mixing of insulin
  - self blood or urine glucose monitoring
  - interpretation of results of self blood or urine glucose monitoring
  - problem shooting skills

4.3 Rights of patients

- inform the patients that his/her health care team should provide:
  - continuing education for patients and their families
  - a treatment plan and self-care targets
  - regular assessment of glycaemic control and physical condition
  - treatment for special problems

4.4 Roles of patients

- patients should be encouraged:
  - to understand the nature of the disease and its treatment
  - to integrate the advice into daily life
  - to be in control of the diabetes on a day-to-day basis
  - to communicate with health care team
  - to adopt a positive attitude towards the disease?

4.5 General aspects of treatment

- aims of treatment:
  - relief of symptoms
  - reduce long-term complications
  - improve quality of life and well-being
  - treatment of associated conditions
- know the targets
  - A: HbA_{1c} <7%
  - B: blood pressure <130/80 mmHg
  - C: LDL-cholesterol <2.6 mmol/l
- **emphasize: blood glucose levels depend on diet, exercise and drugs and can be affected by intercurrent illnesses, stresses and pregnancy** (see 4.6 for causes that can affect glycaemia)
- avoid over-treatment and fluctuations in blood glucose levels in the elderly
- maintain optimal glycaemic control especially in young patients
- control other cardiovascular risk factors, e.g. blood pressure, serum lipid levels, maintain ideal body weight and stop smoking
- emphasize necessity of long-term follow up
- **reinforce: diabetes is a lifelong disease but compatible with an active and healthy lifestyle**

4.6 Factors which interfere with glycaemic control in diabetic patients

1 Meal planning
  - size, composition, timing
2 Exercise
  - intensity, duration, timing
3 Stress
  - diurnal variation
  - emotion, menstruation
  - concurrent illnesses
  - pregnancy

4 Insulin injection
  - depth, angle, site, lipohypertrophy, temperature, exercise
  - unpredictable absorption profile, antibody binding, unstable mixtures
5 Patient error
6 Changes in body weight

4.7 Self-monitoring

- emphasize:
  - optimal glycaemic control is associated with 50–60% risk reduction in the development or progression of microvascular complications in both Type 1 and Type 2 diabetes
  - risk of microangiopathic complications increases sharply when HbA_{1c} exceeds 8.5%
  - **glycaemic control can only be assessed by frequent self-monitoring due to poor correlation between symptoms and blood glucose levels**
  - it is a form of self-education which provides direct feedback to the patients regarding factors that may affect glycaemic control
- unstable Type 1 diabetic patients or when altering treatment in intensively-treated patients:
  - 3–4 tests per day pre-prandially with occasional 3 a.m. and 2 hours post-prandially
- stable Type 1 diabetic patients:
  - pre-prandial daily profile 2 times per week (occasionally 3 a.m. and 2 hours post-prandially)
- stable Type 2 diabetic patients:
  - 3–4 tests (blood or urine) per week pre-prandially and 2 hours post-prandially

4.7.1 Urine monitoring

- the renal threshold for glycosuria averages 10 mmol/l but increases with age and duration of diabetes
- does not distinguish between hypoglycaemia, normoglycaemia and hyperglycaemia
- provides a rough guide for the **trend** of glycaemic control but generally correlates poorly with blood glucose levels

- probably acceptable only in elderly patients with stable diabetes or in those who refuse/fear finger pricking or cannot afford self blood glucose monitoring (SBGM)

4.7.2 Self blood glucose monitoring (SBGM)

- capillary blood glucose values are usually 10% lower than venous plasma glucose concentration
- most SBGM machines generate blood glucose values which are clinically acceptable although the majority tend to under-read by 10–15% compared to venous plasma glucose and the discrepancy increases further with higher values
- taken together, SBGM readings are generally 20% less than venous plasma glucose which is the reference test
- patients should be appropriately educated so that they do not over-correct "low normal" value or feel unduly secure with "high normal" values
- increasingly popular and offers more advantages over urine monitoring:
  - provides direct feedback regarding lifestyle factors (diet, exercise, illness, stress) which affect blood glucose levels
  - helps to confirm or refute hypoglycaemic complaints
  - provides an aid to recognize emergency situations
  - offers a more "real life" profile to facilitate the adjustment of components of treatment regimen, e.g. diet, exercise and drugs, than a "hospital profile"
  - most patients find SBGM useful once educated appropriately
- **SBGM strongly recommended for:**
  - pregnancy
  - unstable diabetes
  - recurrent hypoglycaemia or ketosis
  - hypoglycaemic unawareness
  - abnormal renal threshold
  - intensive insulin therapy (e.g. multiple injections or continuous subcutaneous insulin infusion)
- **SBGM recommended for:**
  - all insulin-treated patients
  - young patients on oral agents
- **increased frequency of self-monitoring required:**

- during times of illness
- in the presence of hypo- or hyperglycaemic complaints
- plan for pregnancy
- change of daily routines (e.g. travelling, increased exercises, missed meals)
- change of therapy

- review and explain the results to the patients
- validate the results by periodically measuring venous plasma glucose and HbA$_{1c}$
- **reasons for erroneous results:**
  - inappropriate techniques
  - falsified results
  - faulty meters

4.7.3 Accessories (test strips and meters)

- Criteria for choosing glucose test strips (urine or blood) and glucose meters include:
  - accuracy
  - consistency
  - user acceptability
  - affordability

4.8 Insulin administration (see also Chapter 7)

4.8.1 Units, types of insulin and syringes

- available concentrations: in developed countries, 100 u/ml (U100) insulin is the standard preparation while 40 u/ml (U40) insulin is still available in many developing countries, hence the need to check the strength of insulin before changing insulin dosages especially in patients who have lived in other countries previously
- 3 types of syringes are available: 0.3 ml, 0.5 ml and 1 ml
- syringes may be re-used by the same patient with recapping of the needles which should be discarded when blunt
- insulin pen has the following advantages — easy to carry, simple to operate, facilitates the administration of multiple injections, suitable for patients with poor vision and the elderly

- different types of insulin [animal (porcine, bovine, highly purified monocomponent) and human] have different modes of actions and should **not** be interchanged without prior consultation with health care providers

4.8.2   Storage of insulin

- should be stored in refrigerator (2–8°C) but away from the freezer; if fridge is not available, keep in sealed pack in water
- storage at room temperature (25–30°C) away from the sunlight is acceptable for a few weeks at most
- discard insulin with clumps or if "discoloured"
- discard frozen insulin
- check expiry date

4.8.3   Insulin mixing

- when mixing insulin, clear neutral regular (short-acting) insulin should be drawn **before** the cloudy isophane protamine (NPH = neutral protamine hagedorn) insulin
- NPH and regular insulin formulations do not interact and may be stored for future use
- zinc suspension insulin (IZS) may delay the actions of the regular insulin after mixing and should be used immediately

4.8.4   Sites of injection

- absorption of insulin is fastest from the abdomen, slowest from the thigh and intermediate from the buttock and arm
- absorption of insulin is increased in exercising limbs and heat exposure
- rotation of insulin injection should be within the same anatomical site (preferably abdomen), avoid switching too frequently from one anatomical site to another
- wipe injection site before injection, alcohol swab not usually required

4.9 Sick day management

4.9.1   In Type 2 diabetes

- unlikely to decompensate in previously stable patients

unless in the presence of significant illnesses (e.g. stroke, myocardial infarction, severe infection)

- continue with oral agents with frequent self-monitoring, e.g. 6–8 hourly especially if food intake is reduced
- should maintain adequate caloric and fluid intake (e.g. liquid/soft diet if anorexic) to avoid hypoglycaemia
- insulin may need to be used temporarily if glycaemic control is inadequate

4.9.2   In Type 1 diabetes

- **diabetic ketoacidosis may rapidly develop in the presence of illness and omission of insulin**
- maintain oral intake with light meal and regular insulin regimen
- avoid dehydration, if vomiting or having diarrhoea, drink water hourly and use sweetened drink if not eating well
- test blood glucose level frequently, e.g. every 2–4 hours, and use supplements of regular insulin, e.g. 5–10 units every 4 hours, to maintain a blood glucose level <14 mmol/l; alternatively, increase daily requirement by 20%
- check for urinary ketones frequently
- contact doctor if
  - urine ketones exceed "traces"
  - persistent vomiting or inability to eat
  - blood glucose levels ≥14 mmol/l or significant deterioration from the "normal" profile of the patient
  - deteriorating general condition

4.10   Hypoglycaemia

- insulin-treated patients (preferably, all diabetic patients) should carry a card or bracelet indicating diagnosis and actions to be taken during severe hypoglycaemia
- rapidly absorbable glucose (e.g. candies, Glucotab) should also be carried

4.10.1   Symptoms

- blood glucose levels ≤ 2.2 mmol/l or symptoms reversed by glucose administration

- in normal subjects, insulin secretion is suppressed when blood glucose <3 mmol/l, this is followed by activation of counter-regulatory hormones when blood glucose level falls below 2.2 mmol/l
- autonomic (due to activation of counter-regulatory hormones especially catecholamines):
  - sweating, palpitations, nausea, fatigue, moody, anxiety, hunger, tremor
  - useful warning symptoms for patient to take corrective actions
  - loss of autonomic symptoms can lead to hypoglycaemic unawareness and rapid deterioration to coma due to long duration of diabetes, concurrent beta blocking drugs and autonomic neuropathy
- neuroglycopenic (due to deprivation of glucose in the central nervous system):
  - failure to concentrate, double vision, perioral numbness, confusion, irrational behaviour and neurological signs especially in the elderly
  - symptoms are subtle and may be missed by patients resulting in rapid loss of consciousness

4.10.2   In patients treated with oral agents

- hypoglycaemia is common and potentially fatal in patients treated with sulphonylureas which have insulinogenic effects
- antidiabetic drugs such as metformin or α glucosidase inhibitors (e.g. acarbose) **alone** do not usually cause hypoglycaemia due to their lack of effects on insulin secretion
- prolonged hypoglycaemia can occur with sulphonylureas and patients should be hospitalized for observation after a significant episode of hypoglycaemia (e.g. coma or requiring assistance from another person)
- risk of hypoglycaemia of sulphonylureas in descending order: glibenclamide > chlorpropamide > gliclazide > glipizide
- the increased risk of hypoglycaemia of glibenclamide is due to its common use and active metabolite (4-OH-glibenclamide) which is renally excreted

4.10.3   In insulin-treated patients

- very common but readily correctable and less prolonged except for long acting insulin
- well-informed patients may not require hospital admission if precipitating cause can be readily identified (e.g. omission of meal, increased physical activity) after the dosage has been adjusted accordingly

4.10.4   Precipitating causes

- **reinforce the interrelationships between blood glucose, diet, exercise and drugs (oral agents or insulin)**
- defective counter-regulation due to impaired glucagon and catecholamine secretion in patients with long duration of disease is the commonest cause of hypoglycaemia in Type 1 diabetes
- other causes:
  - overzealous glycaemic control, e.g. intensive insulin therapy
  - errors of dosage and timing
  - mismatch of meal, medications and exercise
  - exercise (this can be followed by a prolonged period of increased sensitivity due to the replenishment of glycogen storage in muscle from circulating blood glucose)
  - recent weight loss
  - alcohol (especially with empty stomach) due to its inhibitory effect on gluconeogenesis (see 5.2)
  - interaction with drugs which improve glucoregulation or alter pharmacokinetics of antidiabetic drugs
    - beta blocking agents
    - angiotensin converting enzyme (ACE) inhibitor
    - α blocking agents
    - aspirin
  - renal impairment
  - liver disease
  - extremes of ages
  - change of insulin preparations (e.g. animal to human insulin, U40 to U100 insulin)
  - inadvertent intramuscular injection with depot effect

or increased insulin absorption due to changes in injection sites or skin condition
 – changes in injection sites
 – changes in lifestyle or routines (e.g. travelling)
 – failure to reduce insulin dosage in the post-partum or post-infection period or following weight reduction
 – hypoglycaemic unawareness
 – autonomic neuropathy
 – defective counter-regulation due to long duration of diabetes or coexistent diseases, e.g. hypoadrenalism, hypopituitarism
 – psychological problems (deliberate overdosage, manipulative behaviour)
- **old age especially in institutionalized patients and renal impairment are the major causes of drug-induced hypoglycaemia in our local Type 2 diabetic patients**

4.10.5   Treatment of hypoglycaemic symptoms

- if possible, confirm with capillary blood glucose test strip
- 10–15 g equivalent simple glucose for rapid absorption, e.g.
  – 1 glass fruit juice or soft drink
  – 3 heaped teaspoons of sugar
  – 3–5 candies or sweets
  – 2 cubes of glucose tablets (Glucotab, b.d.)
- complex carbohydrates should be taken (e.g. biscuits or sandwiches) to avoid recurrence of hypoglycaemia
- **intravenous glucose is unnecessary if the patient is conscious**
- identify precipitating causes and reduce dosage of treatment accordingly
- reinforce education to prevent recurrence

4.10.6   Treatment of hypoglycaemic coma

- if possible, confirm with capillary blood glucose test strip
- initially 10–25 ml of 50% (50 g per 100 ml) dextrose solution (D_{50}) intravenously followed by infusion of 10% (10 g per 100 ml) dextrose solution (D_{10}) until oral intake is satisfactory
- 1 mg glucagon intramuscularly if no venous access

- monitor blood glucose levels 4–6 hourly
- **abruptly stopping all insulin therapy in a Type 1 diabetic patient following an episode of hypoglycaemia not related to over-treatment may result in hyperglycaemia and even diabetic ketoacidosis**

4.11 Diabetic complications

- explain the nature of diabetic microvascular (retinopathy, neuropathy and nephropathy) and macrovascular complications
- duration of disease and glycaemic control are the main factors for the development of microvascular complications
- genetic factors may be involved in the development of diabetic complications but at present there are no reliable predictive genetic markers
- results of the DCCT (Diabetes Control and Complication Trial) confirm that good glycaemic control reduces the risk of onset and rate of progression of microvascular complications by 60%
- risk of microvascular complications increases sharply if HbA_{1c} exceeds 8%
- weight reduction, cessation of smoking, control of hypertension and hyperlipidaemia, and use of aspirin may have greater impacts on macrovascular complications
- there are also evidence showing that good glycaemic control is associated with improved clinical outcomes in patients with macrovascular complications (e.g. stroke or myocardial infarction)
- advice on foot care (see 8.2)
- **emphasize the preventability of these complications**

4.12 Treatment non-compliance

- 40–50% of patients with chronic diseases such as diabetes mellitus are non-compliant.
- patient factors
  - poor acceptance of one's illness
  - lack of training for the management of the treatment
  - inappropriate interpretation or misconception of one's illness and treatment
  - lack of motivation for long-term treatment

- confusion between internal and external control
- doctor factors
  - medical identity — emphasis on direct intervention (emergency or crisis model)
  - difficulties in listening to the patient
  - over ambitious treatment objectives
  - poor management of treatment relapses
  - poor preparation of the patient to manage his treatment
  - long-term follow up based on somatic problems only
  - non-participation of the patient's family and immediate circle
- illness (diabetes, a classic model)
  - absence of alarm signals — silent disease
  - incurable chronic disease
  - long-term disabling complications
  - discordance between the patient's complaints and the objective signs of the illness

4.13 Psycho-sociological problems

- diabetic child
  - parent's perspective
    - guility feelings; tendency to spoil the affected child; deprivation of love to the siblings; worries over growth retardation and poor academic achievement; feeling a great burden due to the need to acquire new knowledge and skills on caring of diabetes; feeling hurt when giving shots and doing finger pricks; ashamed of having a diabetic child; worries over possibilities of acute and chronic diabetic complications
  - diabetic child's perspective
    - feeling hurt when being pricked; restricted eating and drinking; isolation from other "normal" children
- adolescent
  - poor compliance to diet, drug and self-monitoring; peer influence; poor self-image; worries over future prospect
- adult
  - worries over the disease's effects on job, romance,

marriage, sex, sports; fear of the disease being hereditary; hypoglycaemic unawareness; low self-esteem; worries over possibilities of acute and chronic diabetic complications
- elderly
  - poor compliance because of advanced age; feelings of being a great burden on the family especially when help is needed in giving insulin injections and self-monitoring; poor learner

4.14 Financial aspect

- costs defrayed by a diabetic patient in Hong Kong
  - cost for a medical consultation in a public health care institution ~ HK$44
  - cost for a blood glucose testing machine ~ HK$1,500–1,700
  - cost for a capillary blood glucose H'stix test ~ HK$7
  - cost for a urine glucose test ~ HK$1
  - cost for an insulin syringe ~ HK$1.5
  - cost for diabetic foods?
- in Hong Kong, if a patient is on public assistance, he is entitled to 100% reimbursement from the Medical Social Work department for buying these appliances and additional allowances for extra diet
- in most Asian countries, there is often no provision in medical insurance schemes to cover these costs and most patients have to defray these expenses

Chapter 5

Dietary management and exercise in diabetes mellitus

5. Dietary management and exercise in diabetes mellitus

5.1 Goals of dietary management

- to achieve and maintain optimal glycaemic control
- to achieve optimal plasma lipid concentrations
- to maintain or attain reasonable weight for adults
- to maintain or attain normal growth and development in children and adolescents
- to meet increased metabolic needs during pregnancy and lactation
- to treat acute and prevent long-term complications

5.2 Diet composition

- carbohydrate (4 kcal/g):
    - percentage of energy intake should be individualized based on the patient's eating habits and glucose and lipid goals
    - high in dietary fibre (13–16 g per 1,000 kcal per day) especially soluble fibre
- fat (9 kcal/g):
    - <30% of energy intake
    - <10% saturated fat
    - <10% polyunsaturated fat
    - <10% monounsaturated fat
    - <300 mg cholesterol per day
- protein (4 kcal/g):
    - 10–20% energy (0.8 g per kg of ideal body weight per day)
- alcohol (7 kcal/g):
    - contains calories without adding nutritional benefits, should be avoided in obese subjects
    - avoid sugary alcohol (e.g. sweet sherries, ports and sweet wine) and strong liquor (e.g. vodka, whisky)
    - worsens hypertriglyceridaemia
    - inhibits glycogenolysis and gluconeogenesis
    - may cause spontaneous hypoglycaemia especially in malnourished subjects
    - delays counter-regulation in drug-induced hypo-glycaemia

- diabetic patients treated with oral drugs or insulin should always take snacks in the form of complex carbohydrate with an alcohol binge to avoid hypoglycaemia
- may lead to intoxication and interferes with glycaemic control
- fatal hypoglycaemia can occur when insulin overdose is taken in combination with alcohol
- Salt:
  - recommended daily intake: 7–9 g
  - avoid high salt (sodium) intake especially in hypertensive patients

5.3 *Healthy eating guidelines in diabetes mellitus*

- eat a variety of foods
- eat meals and snacks at regular times each day and avoid skipping meals or snacks
- eat about the same amount of food every day, avoid eating more than needed
- choose foods with high fibre content
  - soluble fibres (lentils, beans, peas, oats, oranges, apples)
  - insoluble fibres (whole wheat bread, wheat bran, all bran or other whole wheat breakfast cereals)
- reduce fat intake, especially saturated fat
  - limit meat/fish portions
  - trim visible fat before cooking
  - avoid meat with hidden fats, e.g. sausages, luncheon meat, beef brisket, canned meat
  - remove fat from soup
  - use less oil in cooking, e.g. use non-stick pan, avoid frying
  - use low fat products, e.g. skim milk, low fat diet yoghurt, low fat cheese or spread
- avoid regular use of food with high sugar content, use sweetener if needed
- use alcohol in moderation, if at all
- some diabetic foods have high fat content, try to minimize or avoid these products. There is no evidence to suggest that these products offer any special advantages

5.4 Food choices for diabetic patients

- free foods:
  - all green leafy vegetables
  - clear unsweetened soup
  - tea and coffee without sugar
  - seasonings: vinegar, pepper, herbs and spices
  - artificial sweeteners, e.g. Equal, Hermesetas, saccharin, Pal Sweet and Balance (see 5.7)
  - diet drinks, low calorie squash
- foods to be consumed in controlled portions:
  - cereals: bread, plain biscuits, rice, pasta
  - meat: lean pork, beef, fish, poultry without skin
  - skim milk and other low fat diary products
  - fruits and unsweetened fruit juices
  - root vegetables such as potatoes, carrot, sweet potatoes and taro
  - beans and bean products
  - nuts
  - seasonings: salt, soy sauce
- foods to be restricted or consumed with dietitians' instructions:
  - sugars and sweets
  - sugary drinks, such as fizzy drinks, packet drinks, Ribena, Lucozade, chocolate milk, condensed milk, and malted drinks (Ovaltine, Milo, Horlick)
  - sweet biscuits and buns
  - cakes
  - tinned foods: tinned meat, tinned fish in oil, tinned soup, tinned fruit in syrup
  - roasted pork, roasted duck, roasted goose, Chinese sausages
  - sauces: oyster sauce, ketchup, salad cream, sandwich spread, jam
  - fatty meat: poultry skin, beef belly, chicken feet, pork trotters, pig/ox tail, fatty spare ribs
  - fried food: crisps, chips, dried fish
  - carbohydrate exchange diet (see Appendix II)

5.5 Eating out guidelines

- follow the same meal timing and portions as home diet

- observe the amount of carbohydrate exchange to be taken for that particular meal
- watch portion sizes
- choose more vegetables
- ask how food are prepared and avoid fried food
- never replace cereals (rice or noodles) with meat or fish
- avoid thick sauces and fatty meat dishes
- choose fresh fruits as dessert

5.6   *Weight control*

- it is often difficult to lose weight and many people regain their previous weight after successful weight reduction; hence **avoidance of obesity in the first place is important**
- weight reduction in obese Type 2 diabetic patients is associated with improvement in glycaemic control, blood pressure, lipid profile, notably, triglyceride and increased insulin sensitivity
- body fat is the main culprit for cardiovascular risk and can be reflected to a certain extent by BMI and WHR
- body weight and waist circumference can be used to assess the progress of weight reduction
- according to the National Diabetes Data Group (NDDG), obesity is defined as BMI ≥ 25 kg/m^2 in women and ≥ 27 kg/m^2 in men
- in Hong Kong Chinese aged less than 65 years, the mean BMI in both men and women are 23 kg/m^2, this increases to 24 kg/m^2 in men and 25 kg/m^2 in women with diabetes or impaired glucose tolerance (IGT)
- there is also progressive increase in all cardiovascular risk factors, e.g. blood pressure, plasma glucose, insulin, lipid and urinary albumin excretion with increasing quartiles of BMI or WHR or waist circumferences
- if ideal body weight cannot be achieved, it is still desirable to achieve a moderate weight reduction between 5 and 10 kg which is associated with beneficial clinical outcomes
- energy requirement depends on body weight, basal metabolic rate and energy expenditure and vary considerably between individuals. On average, for a person with a sedentary lifestyle, e.g. housewife and office workers, the

average caloric intake required to maintain body weight
is 30–36 kcal/kg, i.e. 1,500 kcal for a 50 kg person. A
deficit of 3,500 kcal results in 0.5 kg weight loss, hence a
deficit of 500 kcal per day will result in 0.5 kg weight
loss per week
- aim to lose weight steadily, e.g. 0.5 to 1 kg per week;
  weight loss in excess of 2 kg per week should be avoided
- dietary restriction alone without increased energy expenditure may be accompanied by a downward adjustment
  of the basal metabolic rate and hence a slowing down or
  cessation of further weight loss
- **for effective weight reduction, both dietary restriction
  and increased physical activity are required**
- tips to lose weight:
  - eat balanced meals at regular hours
  - do not eat more than needed, eat small helpings and
    say no to second helping
  - eat slowly to obtain satiety
  - avoid and do not stock convenience foods (e.g. crack-
    ers, biscuits, chocolates, ice cream and crisps)
  - avoid snacks, choose food with low calories and high
    fibre contents which tend to be more filling (e.g.
    vegetables, fruits, high fibre crackers)
  - keep busy to take the mind off food
  - increased energy expenditure by doing regular exer-
    cise and increasing daily activities; simple messages
    such as "eat less" and "walk more" have been shown to
    be useful
  - take coffee or tea without sugar, use sweeteners if not
    possible
  - educate and seek support from family and friends
  - reduce alcohol intake, especially sugary drinks
  - weigh regularly especially after successful weight
    reduction to avoid regain
  - read food labels and know about the ingredients and
    caloric contents of packaged foods

5.7   Sweeteners (alternatives to sugars)

- non-carbohydrate sweeteners may help diabetic patients
  to adhere to meal plans
- replacement of sucrose with low-caloric substitute can

result in a reduction of caloric intake which may be beneficial to some obese Type 2 diabetic patients

5.7.1 Strong sweeteners (low or non-caloric sweeteners)

- intensely sweet, only very small amount is required
- contain few or no calories, suitable for diabetic patients and weight watchers
- non-cariogenic

5.7.1.1 Saccharin

- 30 times sweeter than sucrose
- associated with development of cancer in animal studies
- no evidence that consumption increases the risk of bladder cancer in humans (recommended use: <5 mg/kg/day)
- available as 15 mg per tablet
- gives an unpleasant after-taste which is made worse by cooking

5.7.1.2 Aspartame

- a dipeptide containing aspartic acid and phenylalanine methyl ester
- 200 times sweeter than sucrose
- heat labile, sweetness will be affected by cooking or baking
- has a lighter after-taste than saccharin
- used in sugar free chewing gum, table top sweetener

5.7.1.3 Acesulfame-K

- 150 times sweeter than sucrose
- stable to heat
- has a clean sweet taste
- maintains sweetness over a long shelf life
- can be used with other sweeteners
- used in soft diets and low caloric products

5.7.2 Caloric sweeteners (nutritive sweeteners)

- have the same amount of calories as sucrose (4 kcal/g)
- used mainly as bulking agents in food manufacturing
- major sugar substitutes in the manufacture of special diabetic products

- unlikely to offer significant calorie savings
- specialist diabetic products are of little value in modern dietary management of diabetes

5.7.2.1 Fructose

- a natural sugar found in honey and fruits
- 1.5 times sweeter than sucrose
- should be avoided in patients with hypertriglyceridaemia
- mostly used in baking

5.7.2.2 Sorbitol

- half as sweet as sucrose
- more slowly absorbed and is metabolized in the liver
- consumption of large quantities (>30 g/day) may have laxative effects
- requires additional fat to dissolve and give food a creamy texture, hence products containing sorbitol often have more calories than products containing sucrose
- mostly found in jelly, jam, cookies, chewing gum

5.7.2.3 Mannitol

- commonly used as a bulking agent in powdered food or as a dusting agent for chewing gum
- can cause diarrhoea with excessive consumption

5.7.3 *Commercially available sweeteners*

Brand name	Sweetener used
Hermesetas	saccharin
Hermesetas Gold	acesulfame-K
Equal	aspartame
Pal Sweet	aspartame
Balance	aspartame, acesulfame-K, mannitol

5.8　Exercise

- regular exercise helps to reduce weight and improves insulin sensitivity independent of weight reduction
- **regular** aerobic exercise involving rhythmic movements using major muscle groups (e.g. brisk walking, swimming, cycling, jogging) lasting 20 to 60 minutes, 3–5

times per week is preferable to infrequent but strenuous exercise

- advise patient to choose a form of exercise which can be performed on a regular basis, if not possible, an increase of daily activity in the form of walking or climbing stairs can be recommended
- ensure physical fitness and search for vascular, neurological and retinal complications before advising strenuous exercise
- exercise programmes should be individualized with warm up exercise and gradual increase of intensity
- advise proper footwear particularly in subjects with foot problems
- warn against hypoglycaemia and bring along simple sugar for those taking OHA or insulin
- may require monitoring of blood glucose and adjustment of treatment regimen and/or diet
- no extra food is needed for those diabetics on diet control only

5.8.1 *Insulin-treated patients*

- educate about the action (onset and peak) and duration of insulin
- extra carbohydrate, e.g. 10–20 g can be taken for less vigorous exercise with short duration (e.g. less than 30 minutes)
- adjustment of insulin under professional medical instruction may be required for prolonged and strenuous exercise, e.g.
  - reduce morning (evening) regular insulin by 4–5 units if exercising in the morning (evening)
  - reduce morning intermediate acting insulin by 4–5 units if exercising in the afternoon
- SBGM before and after exercise provides the best guide for adjustment of insulin or diet
- avoid exercising in extreme heat or cold
- absorption of insulin from the abdomen is least affected by exercise
- **exercise will correct mild hyperglycaemia but avoid strenuous exercise if random blood glucose level >15 mmol/l which often indicates an insufficiency of**

insulin action. In Type 1 diabetic patients, supplementary regular insulin (and carbohydrate) will be required to reduce the high blood glucose level before the exercise, otherwise hyperglycaemia may arise due to increased counter-regulatory hormones and may lead to ketoacidosis

- delayed hypoglycaemia due to enhanced insulin absorption and replenishment of glycogen store in muscle from circulating blood glucose can occur after strenuous exercise, supplementary snack and reduction of insulin dosage may be necessary

5.8.2   *Non-insulin treated patients*

- exercise promotes weight reduction due to an increase in energy expenditure
- if performed regularly, exercise increases insulin sensitivity independent of weight loss
- **dietary restriction, weight reduction and increased physical activity are particularly useful in patients with IGT and mild Type 2 diabetes** (e.g. asymptomatic, uncomplicated patients who are mildly overweight with a fasting blood glucose level <10 mmol/l)
- these measures also have beneficial effects on cardio-vascular risk factors such as dyslipidaemia particularly hypertriglyceridaemia and insulin resistance

Chapter **6**

Oral drug treatment for diabetes mellitus

6. Oral drug treatment for diabetes mellitus

- antidiabetic drugs such as metformin and α glucosidase inhibitors (e.g. acarbose) do not have effect on insulin **secretion** and do not cause hypoglycaemia if given alone. This is in contrast to sulphonylureas which enhance insulin secretion and hence may cause hypoglycaemia
- treatment with oral agents should be considered after an adequate period (usually at least 4–6 weeks) of diet and exercise therapy which fail to improve glycaemic control significantly
- treatment with oral drugs may be necessary in patients with high blood glucose (e.g. >20 mmol/l, no ketonuria) or marked symptomatology at diagnosis to allow more rapid relief of symptoms, dosage of oral drugs may need to be reduced at a later stage accordingly
- **oral drugs should never be given to pregnant women and patients with Type 1 diabetes**

6.1 Sulphonylureas

- augment endogenous insulin secretion acutely (by blocking the potassium channel of the pancreatic β cells) and improve insulin sensitivity on a long-term basis (probably due to reduced glucose toxicity)
- **first-line treatment in non-obese Type 2 diabetic patients**

	Total daily dosage	Regimen	Tablet strength
glipizide (Minidiab)	2.5–20 mg	o.d./b.d.	5 mg
gliclazide (Diamicron)	40–320 mg	o.d./b.d.	80 mg
glibenclamide (Daonil)	2.5–20 mg	o.d./b.d.	5 mg
tolbutamide (Restinon)	0.5–2 g	b.d./t.d.s	500 mg
chlorpropamide (Diabinese)	250–500 mg	o.d.	250 mg

- chlorpropamide (Diabinese) is excreted by the kidneys and can cause prolonged hypoglycaemia and other side effects such as syndrome of inappropriate anti-diuretic hormone (SIADH) secretion
- risks of hypoglycaemia with different sulphonylureas in descending order:
  glibenclamide > chlorpropamide > glipizide/ gliclazide > tolbutamide
- the increased risk of hypoglycaemia with glibenclamide is related to its common use and active metabolite (4-OH-glibenclamide) which binds to the pancreatic β cells leading to prolonged insulin release
- risk factors for hypoglycaemia (see also 4.10.4):
  - hypoglycaemic unawareness
  - overzealous glycaemic control
  - extremes of ages
  - renal disease
  - liver disease
  - alcoholism
  - drug interactions (e.g. antidiabetic drugs, beta blockers, aspirin, ACE inhibitors)
  - reduced counter-regulatory responses, e.g. hypo-adrenalism, hypopituitarism
  - long duration of disease with defective counter-regulatory responses
- avoid starting glibenclamide or chlorpropamide in elderly patients but probably unnecessary to change therapy in stable patients on low dose treatment
- all sulphonylureas should be given 15–30 minutes before meal for optimal effects
- a change to another sulphonylurea is unlikely to improve glycaemic control. If control remains poor, consider addition of other antidiabetic drugs or change to insulin therapy
- addition of another sulphonylurea does not improve control and increases the incidence of side effects

6.2 Biguanides (metformin)

- metformin 0.5–3 g daily in b.d. or t.d.s. regimen
- no effect on insulin secretion
- enhances insulin action and improves insulin sensitivity

- reduces peripheral glucose production by inhibiting glycogenolysis and gluconeogenesis
- reduces intestinal absorption of glucose
- improves plasma lipid profile especially hyper-triglyceridaemia
- **first-line treatment in obese Type 2 diabetic patients**
- gastrointestinal side effects (up to 20% of patients) can be minimized by starting with low dose, e.g. 250 mg b.d. and increasing the dosage slowly
- avoid use of metformin in patients with significant   liver, kidney (e.g. plasma creatinine >150 µmol/l) or cardiac diseases and alcoholism due to increased risk of lactic acidosis in these patients
- metformin inhibits the conversion of lactate to glucose and can lead to accumulation of lactate in the presence of increased formation (e.g. hypoxia, alcoholism) or reduced clearance (e.g. renal or liver disease) (see also 12.3)
- **in most cases of metformin-related lactic acidosis, contraindications to its use (renal, hepatic, cardiac or respiratory dysfunction or alcoholism) have been present**
- phenformin is associated with high risk of lactic acidosis but is still available in China and some underdeveloped countries

6.3 Thiazolidinediones (TZD)

- two TZDs are currently available: Rosiglitazone (2–4 mg BD) and pioglitazone (15–30 mg daily)
- the first drug of this class, troglitazone, was withdrawn following reports of severe hepatotoxicity
- mode of action: increase insulin sensitivity and hence glucose uptake by the skeletal muscles, decrease hepatic insulin resistance
- effects mediated through peroxisome proliferators-activated receptor-gamma
- other beneficial effects include: decrease in LDL cholesterol particle size, increase HDL-cholesterol, decrease triglyceride, decrease free fatty acid, decrease carotid intima-media thickness, decrease PIA-1 and fibrinogen, improve endothelial function, decrease visceral fat

- adverse effects include mild weight gain, decrease in haematocrit, oedema
- contraindicated in heart failure and liver disease
- monitor liver function at regular intervals

6.4 Anti-absorptive drugs

Acarbose (50–100 mg t.d.s.)
- a competitive inhibitor of α glucosidase which is the enzyme located in the brush border of small intestinal cells to break down disaccharides to monosaccharides
- delays glucose absorption from the intestines and reduces post-prandial blood glucose and insulin excursion
- **the drug must be taken with the first or second mouthful of food for optimal effects**
- does not cause significant malabsorption but may cause mild weight loss
- reduces HbA_{1c} by 1% compared to placebo in Type 2 diabetic patients treated with diet, oral agents or insulin
- most effective in patients with dietary failure, mild disease and in those with high post-prandial blood glucose levels
- side effects include flatulence and diarrhoea but incidence declines with time
- gradual dose titration may reduce side effects
- abnormal liver function tests have been reported in some patients taking high dosages (e.g. 300 mg t.d.s.)

6.5 Anti-obesity drugs

Most Type 2 diabetic patients are overweight/obese. The excess weight contributes to insulin resistance and hence poor diabetic control. By reducing weight through life-style changes, insulin sensitivity will improve along with glycaemic control. Hence anti-diabetic drugs play a role in the management of obese Type 2 diabetic patients. These drugs, however, must be taken in conjunction with diet modification.

Orlistat (Xenical)
- available as 120 mg capsules to be taken 1–3 times daily regularly or when required
- licenced in use in children (age 12–16 years)

- inhibits intestinal lipase resulting in fat malabsorption (only ~30% of dietary fat will not be absorbed)
- to be taken before meal or within 1 hour after meal
- predominantly exerts its action inside the small intestines with less than 1% systemic absorption
- no significant drug interactions
- effective in weight reduction and prevents progression of IGT to diabetes
- steatorrhoea is the major side-effect which is dependent on diet. Deficiency in fat-soluble vitamins is generally not a clinical problem
- certain anti-diabetic drugs such as metformin and acarbose may need dose reduction to minimize intestinal side-effects

Sibutramine (Reductil)
- available as 10 mg and 15 mg capsules once daily
- a specific serotonin and noradrenaline re-uptake inhibitor
- induces weight by enhancing satiety and increasing thermogensis
- side-effects include dry mouth, constipation, sleep disturbances, increased heart rate and very rarely uncontrolled hypertension
- contraindicated in subjects on psychiatric medications
- short-term studies have shown comparable efficacy as orlistat in patients with Type 2 diabetes

6.6 Oral drug failure (primary or secondary)

- sulphonylureas, biguanides and α glucosidase inhibitors act synergistically and can be given when single agent therapy has failed
- consider the following factors before change to insulin therapy:
  – dietary non-adherence particularly in the obese patients
  – failure to increase level of physical activity
  – consider SBGM to provide feedback and enhance self-care
  – intercurrent illnesses, e.g. tuberculosis, infections and thyrotoxicosis
  – poor treatment compliance (see also 4.12)
  – other medications, e.g. steroids, thiazides (especially in high dosages), which may worsen glycaemic control

- – early insulin treatment may be necessary in non-obese, Type 2 diabetic patients with marked symptoms (primary oral drug failure)
- a period of intensive education together with an understanding of the impending need for insulin may result in improved glycaemic control in 20–25% of such patients
- secondary oral drug failure frequently occurs in Type 2 diabetic patients after long duration of diseases, estimated failure rate is 5–10% yearly
- 50% of Type 2 diabetic patients require insulin treatment for optimal control after 10 years history of illness
- **indiscriminate increase of dosages of oral agents or premature transfer to insulin may result in unpredictable hypo-glycaemia and worsen obesity (particularly in obese patients)**

6.7 Combination therapy of insulin and oral agents

6.7.1 Supplementary insulin treatment

- fasting hyperglycaemia in Type 2 diabetes is often due to non-suppression of nocturnal hepatic glucose production. This may be improved by administration of intermediate or long-acting insulin at bedtime, in addition to oral agents
- in Hong Kong Chinese Type 2 diabetic patients with secondary oral drug failure, low dose supplementary insulin treatment (mean dose: 14 u/day) was associated with a 2% reduction in HbA_{1c} and a weight gain of 2 kg compared with similar glycaemic control but weight gain of 5 kg in patients treated with full-dose insulin replacement regimen (mean dose: 57 u/day)
- supplementary insulin can be used as an "interim" regimen before the patient is switched over to a full-dose insulin regimen. It also allows a smoother transition with easier glycaemic control. Patients often find this combination therapy more acceptable than abrupt cessation of oral drug and transfer to insulin
- combination therapy of bedtime insulin and oral agents in selected patients may reduce insulin requirement and hence, peripheral hyperinsulinaemia, with beneficial effects on weight gain, and possibly blood pressure
- in Chinese Type 2 diabetic patients treated with metformin-sulphonylurea-insulin combination, glycaemic

control can usually be maintained despite a reduction in sulphonylurea dosage. However, withdrawal of metformin results in significant deterioration in glycaemic control, suggesting that metformin has significant synergistic effects with insulin in patients treated with combination therapy of insulin and oral agents

- in Caucasian Type 2 diabetic patients, combination treatment with insulin and metformin is associated with better glycaemic control than that with insulin and sulphonylureas

- start by **supplementing** the existing oral drug regimen with 0.1–0.2 u/kg of intermediate or long acting insulin given at bedtime and increase by 2 units increments at 3–4 daily intervals. If glycaemic control fails to improve with 0.5 u/kg of insulin or more, a full insulin regimen **substituting/replacing** the oral regimen is often needed

6.7.2 Replacement insulin treatment

- combination treatment with insulin and oral agents is more effective in patients with **early** oral drug failure than in patients who have been established on full insulin regimen (see Chapter 7 for regimen and dosage)

Table 6.1 Mode of action of oral antidiabetic drugs

	Insulin secretion	Insulin sensitivity	Carbo-hydrate absorption	Hypo-glycaemia
sulphonylurea	↑↑↑	↑	↔	↑↑
metformin	↔	↑↑↑	↓	↔
thiazolidinedione	↔	↑↑	↔	↔
α glucosidase inhibitor (e.g. acarbose)*	↔	↑	↓↓↓	↔
guar gums or dietary fibres	↔	↑	↓↓	↔

* must be taken with the first few mouthfuls of food
↑ = increase; ↓ = decrease; ↔ = no effect

6.8 Treatment of Type 2 diabetic patients

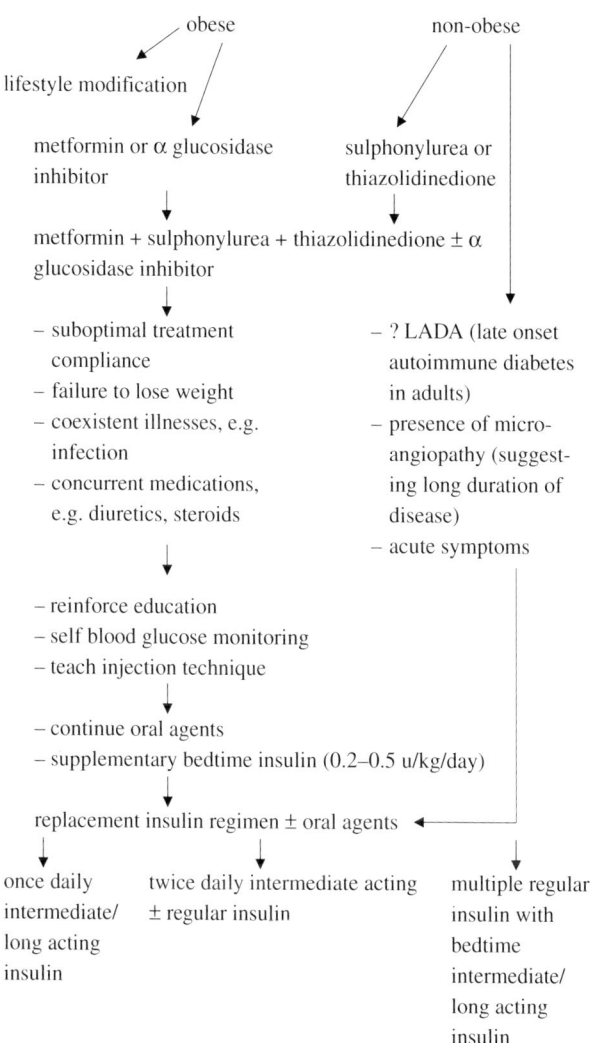

obese   non-obese

lifestyle modification

metformin or α glucosidase inhibitor   sulphonylurea or thiazolidinedione

metformin + sulphonylurea + thiazolidinedione ± α glucosidase inhibitor

– suboptimal treatment compliance
– failure to lose weight
– coexistent illnesses, e.g. infection
– concurrent medications, e.g. diuretics, steroids

– ? LADA (late onset autoimmune diabetes in adults)
– presence of micro-angiopathy (suggesting long duration of disease)
– acute symptoms

– reinforce education
– self blood glucose monitoring
– teach injection technique

– continue oral agents
– supplementary bedtime insulin (0.2–0.5 u/kg/day)

replacement insulin regimen ± oral agents

once daily intermediate/ long acting insulin

twice daily intermediate acting ± regular insulin

multiple regular insulin with bedtime intermediate/ long acting insulin

Chapter **7**

Insulin

7. Insulin

7.1 Indications

- Type 1 diabetes with tendency to develop unprovoked ketosis
- non-obese Type 2 diabetic patients who are severely symptomatic at diagnosis or have primary oral drug failure
- secondary oral drug failure
- transient therapy at times of stress with poor glycaemic control (e.g. infection, peri-operative periods, myocardial infarction, cerebrovascular accident)
- pregnancy when diet alone fails
- optimize glycaemic control with insulin in Type 2 diabetic women planning for pregnancy

7.2 Actions and duration of insulin

- **marked inter-individual and intra-individual variations in the absorption of insulin and sensitivity to insulin, hence the table below only represents a rough estimate of the profiles of actions of these insulin preparations**
- unlike physiological insulin which can be switched "on and off" depending on food intake and prevailing blood glucose levels, administered insulin cannot be "switched off" so that regular meals and activities are desirable to match insulin action (see Figures 7.1a and 7.1b)
- **SBGM offers the best guide for adjustment of the insulin dosage**

	Onset (h)	Peak (h)	Duration (h)
Very short acting (insulin analogue) — clear			
Lispro	immediate	15 mins	1–2
Aspart	immediate	15 mins	1–2
Short acting (neutral regular insulin) — clear			
Actrapid/Humulin-R	0.5	1–2	4–6
Intermediate acting (isophane protamine insulin, NPH) — cloudy			
Protaphane/Humulin-N	1–2	4–8	16–20
Glargine	1–2	peakless	18–20
Long acting (insulin zinc suspension,, IZS) — cloudy			
Monotard/Humulin-L	3–4	6–14	18–24
Very long acting (insulin zinc suspension IZS) — cloudy			
Ultratard/Humulin-UL	4	10–20	30+

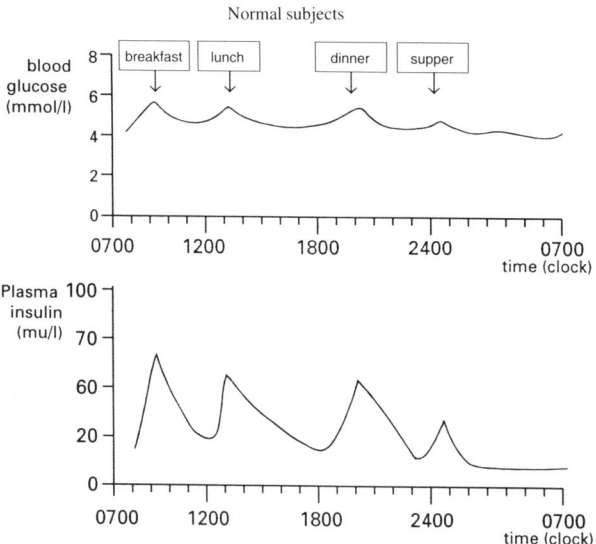

Fig. 7.1a   Blood glucose and plasma insulin concentrations in normal subjects

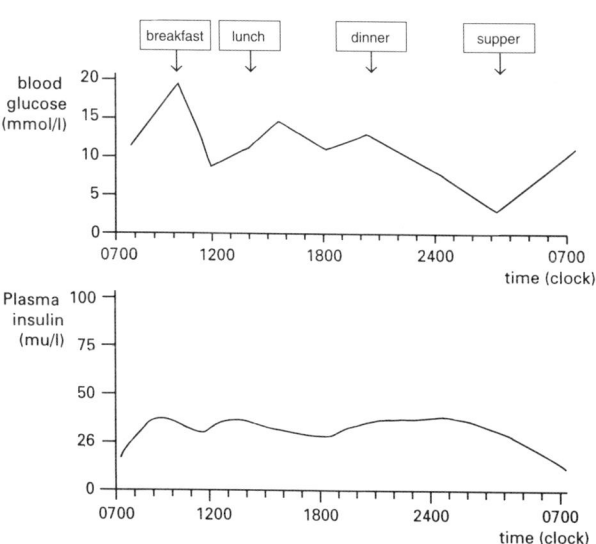

Fig. 7.1b   Blood glucose and plasma insulin concentrations in diabetic individuals

- biphasic insulin, e.g.
  - Mixtard 30/70: 30% Actrapid, 70% Protaphane
  - Humulin 30/70: 30% Humulin-R, 70% Humulin-N
  - other combinations include 40/60, 50/50, 20/80

7.3 Types of insulin

- animal (porcine/beef) insulin — antigenicity can be a problem, now rarely used
- highly purified monocomponent (MC) insulin — animal insulin with removal of most impurities, hence less antigenicity
- human (HM) insulin — prepared either by DNA engineering or biochemical transformation of porcine insulin by substitution of alanine with threonine in position B30, human insulin is now increasingly used and replacing other preparations
- insulin analogue — very short acting insulin with transposition of proline at position 29 with lysine at position 28 in the B chain
  - particularly effective in reducing post-prandial glycaemic excursion and latent hypoglycaemic episodes often with beneficial effects on HbA_{1c}
- peakless insulin — lower post-absorptive plasma glucose and decreases risk of hypoglycaemia

7.4 Regimen (see Figure 7.2)

- once daily dosage
  - for the elderly or patients with advanced disease in whom symptomatic relief is the primary aim or those who refuse more frequent injections
  - intermediate or long acting insulin before breakfast
- twice daily dosage
  - minimal requirements for young patients
  - intermediate acting insulin before breakfast and supper
  - intermediate acting insulin combined with short acting insulin before breakfast and supper
- multiple dosage
  - very long acting or long acting insulin given at bedtime or in the morning with short acting insulin before each meal
  - twice daily very long acting or long acting insulin with short acting insulin before each meal
- continuous subcutaneous insulin infusion (insulin pump)

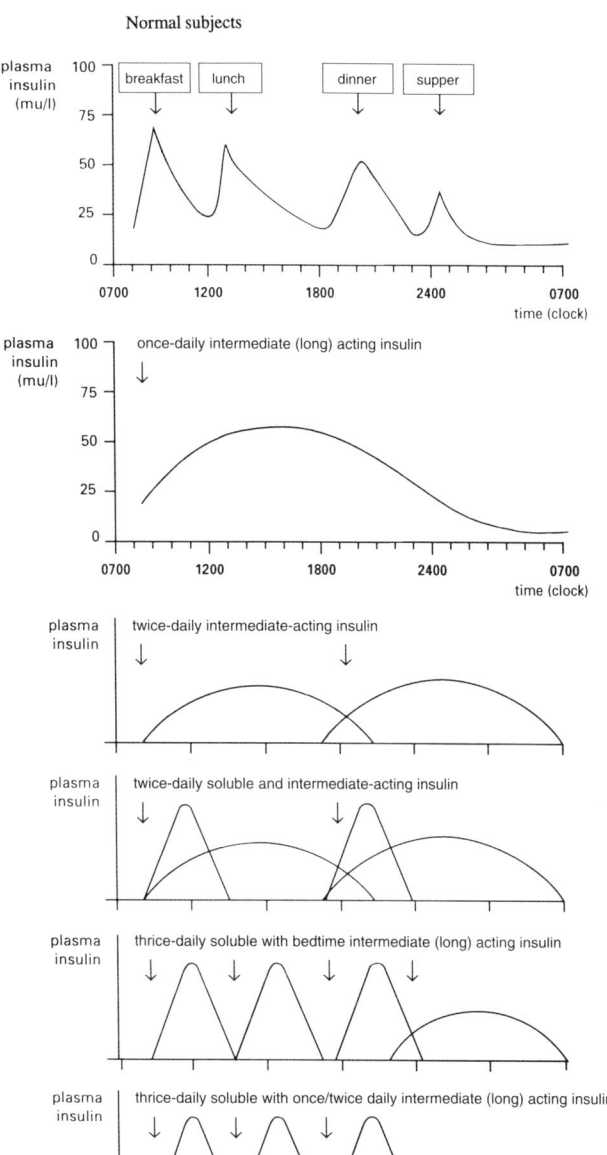

Fig. 7.2 Insulin regimens available in the treatment of diabetic patients

- mimics physiological insulin profile with basal insulin secretion and post-prandial increase
- continuous infusion of regular insulin at pre-set hourly basal rate and boluses at meal time for intensive glycaemic control, e.g. during pregnancy
- allows greater flexibility in lifestyle, e.g. shift work
- allows easier control in patients with brittle diabetes or marked dawn phenomenon (high blood glucose before rising due to increased growth hormone and cortisol)
- improved quality of life in highly motivated patients who must monitor blood glucose at least 4 times per day
- disadvantages include:
  - high acquisition (machines) and maintenance (accessories) costs
  - risks of diabetic ketoacidosis due to pump failure or blockage of catheter
  - skin infection

7.5 Dosage

- subcutaneous regular insulin should be given 15–30 minutes before meal
- Lispro insulin analogue should be given only immediately before meal to avoid hypoglycaemia

7.5.1 Single dose

- a rough estimate for the starting dose of replacement insulin regimen is 0.3–0.5 u/kg per day or 50% of the body weight (i.e. 18–30 u Protaphane or Humulin-N daily in a 60 kg man)
- for supplementary insulin, the starting dose is 0.2 u/kg or 25% of body weight

7.5.2 Divided doses

- if the patient requires divided dosages, then 2/3 of the total daily requirements may be given before breakfast and the remaining 1/3 before the evening meal
  - e.g. Protaphane 20 u a.m., 10 u p.m. or Humulin-N
- if short acting insulin is required, a ratio of 2:1 of

intermediate acting:short acting insulin may be used initially

- subsequent changes of dosage can be made according to the pre-prandial blood glucose levels (and occasionally 2-hr post-prandial) levels
  - e.g. Protaphane or Humulin-N 12 u, Actrapid or Humulin-R 6 u a.m.
    Protaphane or Humulin-N 8 u, Actrapid or Humulin-R 4 u p.m.
    Mixtard 30/70 or Humulin 30/70 18 u a.m., 12 u p.m.
- in general, if the total daily requirement exceeds 60 units, preferably 40 units, the dosage should be divided to reduce the risk of hypoglycaemia due to depot effect and to smooth overall control

7.5.3 Multiple doses

- mimic physiological profile
- offer greater flexibility in terms of diet, exercise and timing of dosage
- made easier with the introduction of various insulin pens and SBGM
- increasingly popular among young and motivated patients,
  - e.g. 30–40% of daily requirement given as long acting insulin at bedtime with the remaining dosage (60%) given before each meal (e.g. 4–8 u Actrapid or Humulin-R via insulin pen 30 minutes before each meal and 12–15 u Ultratard or Humulin-UL at bedtime)
  - reduce episodes of hypoglycaemia especially in patients with irregular patterns of lifestyle (e.g. shift duties) and marked fluctuations of blood glucose (BG) levels but may not improve overall glycaemic control

7.6 Adjustment of dosage

- **a stable dosage is based on a regular meal plan and physical activity**
- further adjustment can be made according to a day profile of BG which reflects the peak action of the insulin:

- pre-breakfast (evening long acting insulin)
- pre-lunch (morning short acting insulin)
- pre-supper (morning long acting insulin)
- bedtime (evening short acting insulin)
- occasionally 3 a.m. (may be staggered between 2 to 6 a.m.) to detect nocturnal hypoglycaemia
- occasionally 2-hr post-prandial (see Fig. 7.2)

- adjust the dosage of the insulin with peak action at the time when pre-prandial BG is taken
- **avoid altering the dosage too frequently, allow 2–3 days for BG profile to stabilize**
- BG can be affected by the caloric and carbohydrate intake and degree of physical activity in relation to the time of blood taking
- adjust in anticipation:
  - increase (reduce) by 2 units increments if increased (less) food intake or decreased (increased) physical activity is planned
- if additional regular insulin is required, administer in relation to food intake (15–30 minutes before meal)
- **frequent BG monitoring is the best guide for adjusting insulin dosage for a given situation**

7.6.1   Once daily regime

- if fasting BG is high, consider increasing the evening long or intermediate acting insulin, **beware of rebound hyperglycaemia due to nocturnal hypoglycaemia which calls for a reduction of evening insulin dosage**
- if there are swings of BG, consider the possibilities of:
  - inadequate action of insulin, multiple dosage regimen (e.g. twice daily) may become necessary
  - rebound hyperglycaemia with periods of hypoglycaemia (with or without symptoms)
  - rebound phenomenon if high HbA$_{1c}$ is associated with low BG (random or fasting), reduction of dosage may be necessary

7.6.2   Twice daily regime

- start with twice daily intermediate acting insulin
- consider addition of regular insulin if BG profile fluctuates

Blood glucose (BG)	Action
a) ↑ pre-lunch BG or ↑ 2-hr post-breakfast BG	add in or ↑ a.m. regular insulin
b) ↑ pre-supper BG	↑ a.m. intermediate acting insulin
c) ↑ bedtime BG or ↑ 2-hr post-dinner BG	add in or ↑ p.m. regular insulin
d) ↑ pre-breakfast BG	↑ p.m. or bedtime intermediate acting insulin

- reduce dosage accordingly for low BG
- **lowering the fasting BG often improves the overall control for the rest of the day**
- BG level can also be affected by the caloric intake of the meal prior to the injection (e.g. amount of breakfast or mid-morning snack with high pre-lunch BG) or the energy expenditure in the preceding few hours as well as other factors such as site of injection
- **regular snacks between main meals to avoid hypo-glycaemia or excessive post-prandial blood glucose excursion, i.e. frequent small meals**

7.6.3 *Multiple dose regime*

- adjust dosage of regular insulin according to carbohydrate intake
- ↑ short acting insulin according to the pre-prandial BG
- perform 2-hr post-prandial BG occasionally to assess peak action of insulin if control is unsatisfactory
- ↑ long acting insulin given at night if BG on rising is high

7.6.4 *Rebound hyperglycaemia and dawn effects*

- high fasting BG may be due to:
  - **dawn effect:** inadequate action of the long/inter-mediate acting insulin given the night before
  - increased requirement of insulin due to increased counter-regulatory hormones especially growth hormone and cortisol released before rising (e.g. between 3–4 a.m. and 7–8 a.m.)
  - **rebound hyperglycaemia:** rebound hyperglycaemia

following asymptomatic hypoglycaemia at night which evokes a surge of counter-regulatory hormones
- suspect nocturnal hypoglycaemia if patients complain of headache on rising, nightmares, sweating or hunger at night
- bedtime snack is important in patients who have long/intermediate acting insulin at supper or bedtime
- occasionally switching the timing of administration of the long/intermediate acting insulin from dinner to bedtime may reduce episodes of nocturnal hypoglycaemia (the peak of action will be delayed to morning, e.g. 5–7 a.m. rather than in the middle of the night, e.g. 2–3 a.m.)
- **distinguish between dawn effect and rebound hyperglycaemia by performing SBGM at 3 to 4 a.m. (↑ insulin if high BG, ↓ insulin if low BG)**

7.7 Travelling

- when crossing time zones
  - perform frequent SBGM, at 4–6 hourly, especially preprandially and give additional regular insulin 5–10 u 30 minutes before meals to maintain BG <14 mmol/l
  - avoid prolonged period of fasting
- bring medications, diabetes travel kit, and medical certificate
- may keep to origin time zone routine during travel and switch to new time zone routine after arrival
- resume previous regimen when the new routine is stabilized

Chapter 8

Diabetic complications

8. Diabetic complications

- **results of the Diabetes Control and Complications Trial (DCCT) which lasted for 7 years involving more than 1,400 Type 1 diabetic patients indicate that a difference of 2% in HbA_{1c} between those treated intensively with multiple injections or insulin pump and frequent SBGM and consultations (7%) and those treated conventionally with twice daily injections and routine visits (9%) was associated with a delay of onset of retinopathy by 76%, nephropathy, 44%, neuropathy, 69% and a reduction in the progression of retinopathy by 63%, nephropathy, 54% and neuropathy, 60%**
- a prospective study involving Japanese Type 2 diabetic patients treated with insulin also shows similar results
- there is also evidence showing that good glycaemic control improves clinical outcomes in Type 2 patients with history of stroke and myocardial infarction
- the effects of optimal glycaemic control on primary prevention of macrovascular complications are being examined in the UK Prospective Diabetes Study although the general consensus is that intervention improves the outcomes of diabetic patients
- there is experimental evidence showing that chronic hyperglycaemia is associated with alteration of intracellular metabolic pathways and formation of advanced glycation end-products which can lead to tissue damage

8.1 Ophthalmic complications

- diabetic eye complications (mostly retinopathy and cataract) are the leading causes of blindness in industrialized countries, especially in young people
- diabetic subjects are 25 times more at risk for blindness due to retinopathy than the general population
- **over 60% of cases of diabetes-related blindness can be prevented if appropriate treatment is delivered**

8.1.1 Recommended procedures for screening

- obtain clinical data including onset of visual symptoms

and history of glaucoma, cataract and its extraction
- document best visual acuity (unaided, corrected by glasses or pinhole)
- pupil dilatation with 2.5% phenylephrine or tropicamide (0.5 or 1%) eyedrops (one drop in each eye and wait for 10 minutes before examination) in patients with no history of glaucoma or intra-ocular pressure <20 mmHg
- lens examination for cataract with +10 lens in ophthalmoscopy
- fundus examination by direct ophthalmoscopy or retinal photography
- significant retinopathy is uncommon in prepubertal children and in Type 1 diabetic patients with less than 5 years of disease
- due to the preponderance of Type 2 diabetes and considerable overlap in clinical presentation between Type 1 and Type 2 diabetes in Chinese, screening is recommended at diagnosis and at least 2-yearly thereafter
  - 30% of Type 2 diabetic patients have retinopathy at presentation
  - perform yearly examination if diabetic retinopathy appears or more frequently if deemed necessary
  - **more frequent examinations are required during intercurrent illness, in patients with hypertension or renal impairment and during pregnancy**

8.1.2 *Features of diabetic eye disease*

- **sight-threatening diabetic retinopathy requiring immediate referral:**
  - a) **proliferative retinopathy:**
    - new vessels on the optic disc or elsewhere in the retina
    - pre-retinal haemorrhage
    - fibrous tissue
  - b) **advanced diabetic eye disease:**
    - vitreous haemorrhage
    - fibrous tissue
    - recent retinal detachment
    - rubeosis iridis (may lead to glaucoma)
- **early referral**
  - a) **preproliferative retinopathy**

  - venous irregularities (beading, loop, reduplication)
  - multiple haemorrhages
  - multiple cotton wool spots
  - intra-retinal microvascular abnormalities
 b) **non-proliferative retinopathy with macular involvement (maculopathy):**
  - reduced visual acuity not corrected by pinhole (suggestive of macular oedema)
  - haemorrhages and/or hard exudates within one disc diameter of the macula with or without visual loss
  - large circinate or plaque hard exudates within the major temporal vascular arcades
- **routine referral**
 a) **non-proliferative retinopathy**
  - cotton wool spots in small numbers not associated with preproliferative lesions
  - occasional haemorrhages and/or microaneurysms ("dots and blots") and hard exudates not within 1 disc diameter of the macular areas
  - **observe** — few dots and blots in **one** eye only

8.1.3   Management

- referral to specialist for assessment
  - detection of retinopathy
  - visual deterioration uncorrected by pinhole (e.g. >20/70 on Snellen's chart)
  - patients with over 10 years of diabetes
- the use of fluorescein angiography may help to identify neovascularization and delineate areas of retinal capillary non-perfusion
- indirect photocoagulation of ischaemic retina, direct focal photocoagulation of lesions (e.g. microaneurysms, new vessels, etc.), vitrectomy can be offered to patients with different stages of diabetic retinopathy and have been proven to substantially reduce blindness if delivered early
- improved glycaemic control, adequate control of blood pressure, cessation of smoking are also important in the management of diabetic eye disease

8.2 Diabetic foot

- common problem (10% in well controlled patients and

over 70% in poorly controlled patients after 25 years of diabetes)
- patients with somatic (focal neuropathy and distal symmetrical polyneuropathy) and autonomic neuropathy are prone to develop diabetic foot complications
- vascular occlusion, neuropathy and infection markedly increase the risk of ulcer and amputation
- up to 50% of lower extremity amputation in diabetic patients could be prevented if proper education and regular assessment have been conducted

8.2.1 Diabetic foot ulceration

- usually occurs after trauma in the presence of diabetic neuropathy and/or peripheral vascular disease
- diabetic somatic neuropathy:
  - decreased pain sensation increases the risk of trauma
  - decreased proprioception and small muscle wasting lead to altered pressure loading onto the foot
- diabetic autonomic neuropathy:
  - autonomic "autosympathectomy" may result in warm foot due to altered blood flow regulation and dry skin
  - skin cracks and fissures easily occur due to absent sweating
- peripheral vascular disease:
  - foot ischaemia increases proneness to ulceration although pure ischaemic ulcer is uncommon, most diabetic foot ulcers are caused by neuropathy with or without ischaemia
- classification:
  - grade 0: "at-risk" foot, no ulcer
  - grade 1: superficial ulcer, usually under high pressure areas
  - grade 2: deep ulcer, subcutaneous tissue is involved usually with local infection but no bone involvement
  - grade 3: infected ulcer with osteomyelitis and/or abscess formation
  - grade 4: local gangrene of the toes, forefoot or heel
  - grade 5: gangrene of the whole foot

8.2.2 Prevention of diabetic foot problems

- identification of patients with "at-risk" foot is the essence

- patients without risk factors should receive education of foot care and annual clinical assessment
- patients with risk factors should be assessed more frequently and treated promptly
- risk factors include:
  - past history of ulcers or amputation
  - established neuropathy, peripheral vascular disease
  - deformity (claw feet, hammer toes, bunions)
  - skin changes (healed ulcers, acute ulcers, gangrene, dry skin, fissures, fungal infection)
  - peripheral oedema
  - elderly
  - long duration of diabetes
  - poor glycaemic control
  - hypertension
  - smoking
  - hyperlipidaemia

8.2.3   Education of foot care

- diabetic patients must have their feet examined regularly especially in the presence of risk factors (8.2.2)
- avoid extreme temperature, e.g. avoid use of heating pads, test bath water
- appropriate shoes (avoid wearing the same shoes for 4 hours or more, avoid high heels in women, avoid walking barefooted)
- proper exercise (avoid jogging and strenuous walking, cycling and swimming preferred)
- daily examination of the feet for skin changes, ulcers and deformity (use a mirror to examine the plantar surface) especially in high risk patients
- toenails should be trimmed straight across, never cut down the sides of the nails and avoid the use of sharp objects
- prompt treatment of "break" in the skin with redness, swelling, drainage or pain
- seek medical advice regarding the use of potent chemicals including iodine, peroxide or magnesium sulphate and tape adhesives
- avoid chemical skin loosener, salicylic acid preparations

and corn plasters for hyperkeratosis due to their caustic actions and large areas of skin can be broken down
- seek help from podiatrist or trained personnel for corns and callus

8.2.4 *Clinical assessment of diabetic foot*

- shoes:
  - examine if they are ill fitting or worn out
  - examine for foreign bodies
- hygiene:
  - are the feet clean?
  - are the nails trimmed correctly?
  - look between the toes for corns, fissures, fungal infection
- sensation:
  - enquire for symptoms (e.g. numbness in glove and stock distribution)
  - test for large fibre function:
    - vibratory perception using 256 Hz and 128 Hz tuning forks and/or deep tendon reflexes
    - light touch using monofilaments
    - position sense
  - test for smaller fibre function:
    - temperature or pain perception thresholds
- vascular:
  - enquire for symptoms of intermittent claudication
  - palpation of foot pulses (posterior tibial and/or dorsalis pedis)
  - doppler examination — a normal ankle to brachial systolic blood pressure ratio (A/B ratio) should exceed 1, a ratio <0.9 indicates impaired blood flow, a ratio 0.5–0.7 confirms the presence of peripheral vascular disease, a ratio <0.5 suggests that the leg is at risk of complications including amputation
  - if foot pulses are absent, examine proximal pulses (popliteal, femoral) to determine level of occlusion
  - referral to vascular surgeon for further assessment
- imbalance of foot muscles frequently results in deformities (e.g. claw toes, hammer toes) and heel spurs, calluses, cracks and corns which need to be treated by skilled personnel such as podiatrists

8.2.5   Treatment

- diabetic foot, once established, is difficult to treat; hence, **prevention is the essence**
- physiotherapy for improvement of gait disturbances due to pain or muscle imbalance
- daily living devices may improve function in some patients with severe somatic neuropathy
- foot ulcer:
  - deep swabs from the ulcer base to rule out infection
  - X-ray foot to exclude osteomyelitis if suspicious
  - broad spectrum antibiotics for local infection
  - avoid further trauma, pressure or irritation to the wound
  - optimize glycaemic control
  - grade 3 or more severe ulcers need hospital admission
  - surgical debridement, intravenous antibiotics and tight glycaemic control (may need intravenous insulin) are required
  - orthopaedic and/or vascular surgical opinion may be indicated especially in grade 4 or 5 ulcers
  - **after care** is essential to prevent recurrent ulceration

8.3 Diabetic neuropathy

- good glycaemic control prevents the onset of neuropathy and improves symptoms
- exact pathogenesis is uncertain
- possible factors include:
  - ischaemic infarct
  - metabolic toxicity (e.g. sorbitol accumulation in nerve cells)

8.3.1   Diabetic autonomic neuropathy

- parasympathetic damage (failure of heart rate or R-R interval on ECG to increase in response to posture or breathing manoeuvre) occurs early, followed later by sympathetic damage (marked fall of blood pressure with posture or failure to increase with exercise)

- mild, symptomatic postural hypotension ≥11–20 mmHg may respond to elastic stockings while severe and symptomatic patients with postural hypotension ≥30 mmHg may require treatment with fludrocortisone 0.1–0.3 mg daily. Patients may be asymptomatic despite marked fall in blood pressure and do not need treatment
- gastroparesis may respond to antispasmodics, e.g. metoclopramide 10 mg t.d.s. and cisapride 5 mg t.d.s to 10 mg q.i.d.
- diarrhoea and constipation may improve with treatment with bulk forming agents and/or antispasmodics
- troublesome, excessive sweating may be helped by anticholinergic drugs although this is rarely needed
- drugs such as thiazides and beta blockers may aggravate impotence which usually improves with adjustment of therapy. Psychological impotence may be improved by counselling. Physical impotence due to vascular and/or neurological damage may be improved by external vacuum therapy, penile injection or surgical implant, referral to urologist specialized in this area is recommended
- patients with bladder dysfunction and urinary retention should be encouraged to void every 3 to 4 hours during the day, if necessary, using manual suprapubic pressure. Long-term chemotherapy may be required for recurrent urinary tract infections. Operation or long-term catheterization may be required for severe cases with obstructive uropathy

8.3.2   Diabetic peripheral neuropathy

- increases risk of developing foot complications
- improved glycaemic control may significantly improve symptoms if patients present early
- topical application of capsaicin (0.025–0.075% q.i.d.) may improve superficial pain or discomfort
- deep pain may respond to treatment with tricyclic antidepressants (e.g. imipramine 50–150 mg or amitriptyline 25–75 mg nocte ± mexiletine 150 mg o.d.) or carbamazepine (100 mg b.d.)
- amitriptyline will work within days, if no improvement after 4–5 days of treatment, discontinue the drug

- mexiletine, an anti-arrhythmic agent, should be used with caution
- muscle pain may be improved by stretching exercises, skeletal muscle relaxant, non-steroidal anti-inflammatory agent, the latter should be used with caution in patients with renal impairment or taking concurrent angiotensin converting enzyme inhibitor (ACEI) or diuretics or in the elderly

8.3.3 Diabetic amyotrophy and mononeuritis multiplex

- present as quadriceps wasting (amyotrophy) or isolated 3rd or 6th nerve palsy (mononeuritis multiplex)
- usually good prognosis with recovery within weeks to months
- exclude other causes, e.g. intracranial lesions for cranial nerve palsy
- no specific therapy

8.4 Microalbuminuria and renal involvement

8.4.1 Definitions

- about 50% of protein in the urine is albumin, others include tubular proteins and enzymes
- a normal subject excretes 30 mg or less of albumin (normoalbuminuria) in his/her urine daily which may increase at times of stress, exercise or febrile illness
- **clinical proteinuria (positive albustix) indicates an urinary albumin excretion ≥ 300 mg/day (macroalbuminuria) and in the absence of infection or other non-diabetes related causes, is associated with established nephropathy in Type 1 diabetes (and possibly Type 2 diabetes) and likely deterioration in renal function**
- microalbuminuria is a state in which the patient excretes between 30 and 300 mg/day, i.e. an abnormality not detectable by routine albustix
- the prevalence of microalbuminuria is approximately 20–30% in Type 1 diabetes and up to 50% in Type 2 diabetes depending on race

8.4.2   Significance of microalbuminuria

- Type 1 diabetes — a marker for the onset of established diabetic nephropathy and increased cardiovascular risks
- Type 2 diabetes
  - associated with increased risk of cardiovascular death and morbidity
  - over 30% of patients have other causes for increased albuminuria, e.g. renal calculi, glomerulone-phritis
  - its predictive role for the deterioration in renal function in Type 2 diabetes is less certain than in Type 1 diabetes
  - in Chinese, a random spot urine albumin: creatinine ratio ≥5.4 mg/mmol predicts early mortality and deterioration in renal function
- associated with early mortality in apparently healthy elderly

8.4.3   Documentation of microalbuminuria

- **urinary albumin excretion has marked day-to-day intra-individual variations of approximately 50%**
- due to this marked intra-individual variability, micro-albuminuria should be defined using at least 2 samples within 6 months
- collection methods:
  - spot urine albumin/creatinine ratio (mg/mmol) in
    a) random sample
    b) early morning sample (to eliminate the effect of ambulation)
  - a spot urine sample is recommended for screening followed by a timed collection
  - microalbustix strip test is convenient but has less optimal sensitivity and specificity compared to laboratory method
  - timed collections:
    c) 24-hr urinary albumin excretion (UAE) (mg/day)
    d) urinary albumin excretion rate (AER) (μg/min) over a timed period, e.g. 4 hours
    e) timed early morning urine (μg/min)
       - record time of going to bed and on rising
       - complete collection of urine sample during the timed period

8.4.4   Range of values

Table 8.1   Screening for microalbuminuria in diabetic patients

Collection method	Measurements	Units
Screening test (Spot urine sample)		
random or early morning	albumin concentration	<20 mg/l
	albumin:creatinine ratio (ACR)	<2.5–3.5 mg/mmol
Confirmatory tests (timed collections)		
4-hr	albumin excretion rate (AER)	20–200 µg/min
24-hr	urinary albumin excretion (UAE)	30–300 mg/day

* definition should preferably be based on two out of three sterile urine collections within a 6-month period

8.4.5   Prevention and treatment of diabetic renal disease

- **rule out other non-diabetes causes of renal failure, especially in the absence of retinopathy or evidence of microangiopathic complications or presence of microscopic haematuria, e.g.**
  - infection
  - calculi
  - co-existing glomerulonephritis (especially microscopic haematuria)
- perform
  - urine microscopy and culture
  - ultrasound scan of the kidneys
  - if indicated, renal biopsies to rule out other non-diabetes related causes
- if UAE <30 mg/day, re-test yearly
- perform renal function test if UAE ≥30 mg/day

Plasma creatinine (µmol/l)	Actions
120–200	repeat 1–2 times yearly
200–300	joint care with renal team
>300	prompt referral to renal team

- **refer patients with established renal disease to the**

appropriate regional renal clinic for assessment of suitability of long term renal replacement

- improvement of glycaemia, adequate control of blood pressure (aim at ≤ 135/85 mmHg) and low protein diet (0.4–0.6 g/kg) have been shown to reduce the rate of deterioration in renal function

- **ACEI has been shown to reduce microalbuminuria and slow the rate of decline of renal function in Type 1 diabetic and in normotensive, microalbuminuric Type 2 diabetic patients with plasma creatinine <200 μmol/l**

- treatment with ACEI is associated with a lower incidence of cardiovascular deaths in hypertensive Type 2 diabetic patients than those treated with calcium channel blockers

- **additional antihypertensive agents such as low dose diuretics and calcium channel blocker are often required for effective BP control in Type 2 diabetic patients**

- cautious use of ACEI and dose titration are required especially in patients with
  - impaired renal function (e.g. plasma creatinine > 150 μmol/l)
  - disproportionately high plasma K^+ suggestive of hyporeninaemic hypoaldosteronism
  - a salt-depleted state (e.g. concurrent use of diuretics in high dosages)
  - possible renal artery stenosis (e.g. absent pedal pulses, renal bruit)
  - concurrent therapy with non-steroidal anti-inflammatory drugs

- check electrolytes 1–2 weeks after commencement of ACEI especially in high risk patients (see above), a small rise in plasma creatinine concentration (10–20%) may be due to acute haemodynamic changes. This may stabilize at a later stage or improve with a reduction of dosage of diuretics if prescribed simultaneously

- a sharp increase in plasma creatinine concentration, e.g. >20% increase, soon after introduction of ACEI raises the possibility of renal artery stenosis or dependency on angiotension II for autoregulation of renal blood flow, the use of ACEI should be used with extreme caution in these patients

- renal replacement therapy (peritoneal or haemodialysis) or renal transplantation are the only treatments available for end stage renal failure
- **moderate renal impairment not requiring dialysis is associated with increased risk of cardiovascular death and morbidity and poor quality of life**

Chapter **9**

Diabetes mellitus and hypertension

9. Diabetes mellitus and hypertension

- **co-existing hypertension accelerates diabetic complications (in particular retinopathy and renal impairment) and atherosclerosis**
- in Type 1 diabetic patients, hypertension usually accompanies and correlates with the severity of nephropathy
- relationship between hypertension and renal disease is less well defined in Type 2 diabetes
- hypertension is present in about 50% of Type 2 diabetic patients and may or may not be accompanied by renal damage
- multiple antihypertensive drugs are often required for adequate control of BP (<135/85 mmHg) in diabetic patients

9.1 Choices of treatment

- non-pharmacological measures, including weight reduction and regular exercise, are particularly useful in patients with mild hypertension (as for mild diabetes and hyperlipidaemia)
  - a) β blockers
    - complex effects on carbohydrate and lipid metabolism, increase TG and TC levels and may precipitate diabetes in predisposed subjects (e.g. obesity)
    - $β_1$-selective agents, e.g. metoprolol, atenolol may be given for cardioprotective effects in patients with unstable angina or myocardial infarction with periodic monitoring of metabolic indices
    - new vasodilating, highly cardioselective β blockers, e.g. celiprolol may be preferred for its more favourable effect on lipid profiles
    - non-selective β blockers (e.g propranolol) should probably be avoided due to increased risk of hypoglycaemic unawareness and delayed counter-regulation
  - b) diuretics
    - may worsen glycaemic control when given in high dosages especially in the presence of hypokalaemia which inhibits insulin release

- may worsen lipid profile with ↑ TG and TC levels
- once daily regimen may improve compliance especially in the elderly with mild disease (monitor electrolytes, glycaemic and lipid parameters regularly)
- e.g. **indapamide 1.25–2.5 mg o.d.**
  bendrofluazide 2.5–5 mg o.d.
  hydrochlorothiazide 12.5 mg–25 mg o.d.

c) calcium channel blocking agents (CCB)
- potent antihypertensive agents with or without anti-anginal properties
- vasodilating and natriuretic effects
- minimal effects on metabolic profile
- side effects such as flushing and oedema occur in 10% of patients and may lead to treatment discontinuation
- variable effects on renal haemodynamics:
- dihydropyridine CCB, e.g. nifedipine dilate both afferent and efferent arterioles and may increase protein-uria despite reducing BP
- non-dihydropyridine CCB such as verapamil and diltiazem dilate efferent arterioles preferentially and may reduce proteinuria more effectively
- the use of short acting CCB such as nifedipine capsule should be discouraged since this may be associated with activation of the neurohormonal systems
- e.g. **amlodipine 5–10 mg o.d.**
  nifedipine retard 20–40 mg b.d
  nifedipine GITs 30–60 mg o.d.
  felodipine 5–10 mg o.d.
  diltiazem 30 mg t.d.s. to 90 mg t.d.s.
  isradipine SR 5–10 mg o.d.

d) angiotensin converting enzyme inhibitors (ACEIs)
- minimal effects on metabolic profile
- improve insulin sensitivity, glycaemic control and hypertriglyceridaemia
- reduce mortality and cardiovascular morbidity in patients with post-myocardial infarction and Type 2 diabetic patients with hypertension
- improve ventricular function especially in patients

with clinical heart failure or ejection fraction <45%

– reduce proteinuria in Type 1 and Type 2 diabetic patients

– renoprotective in Type 1 diabetic, and normotensive Type 2 diabetic patients with preserved renal function (plasma creatinine <200 μmol/l)

– renoprotective in non-diabetic patients with renal impairment

– blood pressure lowering effects may be attenuated in patients with salt retention or on a high salt intake

– cough, probably due to accumulation of kinins which are normally degraded by ACE, is a common side effect (20–30%) among local Chinese but treatment discontinuation only occurs in <5% of patients

– increased risk of renal impairment in the presence of:
  • a salt-depleted state (e.g. on high dose diuretics)
  • renal artery stenosis (caution: if absent pedal pulses or renal bruit)
  • interacting drugs, e.g. non-steroidal anti-inflammatory agent, K^+ sparing diuretics

– check serum K^+ and renal function before and 1–2 weeks after initiation of treatment especially in patients with pre-existing renal impairment or disproportionately high plasma K^+

– e.g. **enalapril 2.5–20 mg o.d.**
     perindopril 4–8 mg o.d.
     captopril 6.25 mg–25 mg b.d./t.d.s.
     lisinopril 10 mg –20 mg o.d.
     ramipril 1.25–10 mg o.d.
     quinapril 5–40 mg o.d.
     cilazapril 2.5–5 mg o.d.
     fosinopril 10–40 mg o.d. (only ACEI with dual hepatic and renal elimination)

e) α_1 adrenoceptor blocker
  – minimal effect on metabolic profile
  – may improve lipid profile but no long-term data on clinical end points

- e.g. **prazosin 0.5 mg–5 mg b.d./t.d.s**
  doxazosin 1–16 mg o.d.
  terazosin 1–10 mg o.d.

f) angiotension II (AII) receptor blocker
   - orally active nonpeptide antagonist at the AII type 1a receptors which mediate most of the pathophysiological effects of AII
   - fundamentally a different class of agent but share similar effects with ACEI in experimental studies, yet without the effects due to accumulation of kinins, hence no increased incidence of cough
   - reduce blood pressure effectively and have independent anti-proteinuric effects and cardio-protective effects in elderly patients with heart failure, and patients with LVH
   - long-term renal protection is well-established

- the agents of choice in Type 2 diabetes are ACEIs, ARBs calcium channel blockers, low dose diuretics and α_1 blockers

- combination treatment with ACEIs and CCB or low dose diuretics may be considered in patients with significant hypertension and microalbuminuria, especially in young patients who are going to have long duration of disease

- **familiarize with one or two drugs in each class and consider cost-effectiveness in the choice of treatment**
  - e.g. **losartan 50–100 mg o.d.**
    irbesartan 150–300 mg o.d.
    telmisartan 40–80 mg o.d.
    valsartan 80–160 mg o.d.
    candesartan 8–16 mg o.d.
    olmesartan 10–40 mg o.d.

9.2 *Management of hypertension and proteinuria in diabetic patients*

screening for microalbuminuria in sterile urine

negative	positive

- screen yearly
- optimize risk factors (e.g. body weight, blood pressure,, blood glucose and lipid)

if microalbuminuria persists

ARB or ACEI ± other antihypertensive drugs

- aim at BP <130/80 mmHg
- monitor renal function test (RFT) especially in patients with:
  - impaired RFT (plasma Cr > 150 mmol/l)
  - high plasma potassium
  - concomitant diuretic therapy especially in high dosages
  - evidence of atherosclerosis (e.g. peripheral vascular disease, renal bruit)

- repeat RFT and spot urine albumin every 6–12 months

9.3 Use of antihypertensive agents in diabetic patients

Antihypertensive drug	Clinical benefits	Potential adverse effects/drawbacks
ACE inhibitors	• improves insulin resistance • improve lipid profile • cardioprotective • antiproteinuric • renoprotective	• caution in patients with salt depletion,, hyperkalaemia, renal impairment or renal artery stenosis • variable antihypertensive actions as monotherapy in Type 2 diabetic patients • high incidence of cough
angiotensin II receptor blockers	• beneficial effects as ACE inhibitors in short-term studies • good tolerability profile • low incidence of cough • antiproteinuric • beneficial in patients with LVH and nephropathy	• caution in patients with hyperkalaemia

thiazide diuretics	• proven to reduce cardiovascular disease related mortality and morbidity in hypertension with or without diabetes	• adverse effects especially with high dose treatment
		  – hypokalaemia
		  – worsen glucose tolerance
		  – increase triglyceride levels

Antihypertensive drug	Clinical benefits	Potential adverse effects/drawbacks
β blocking agents	• proven to reduce cardiovascular disease related mortality and morbidity in essential hypertension and post-myocardial diabetic patients	• potential adverse effects on insulin secretion and action • may mask hypoglycaemic symptoms • aggravate peripheral vascular disease, erectile dysfunction
calcium channel blocking agents	• potent antihypertensive agents • some have additional properties (e.g. anti-anginal, antiarrhythmic) • neutral effects on metabolic indices	• no data on clinical endpoints • reports of increased risk of adverse events such as gastrointestinal bleeding, neoplasm and cardiovascular mortality although conclusive evidence is lacking
α blocking agents	• improve insulin resistance • improve lipid profile	• no data on clinical endpoints
vasodilators (e.g. hydralazine)	• reduce blood pressure	• reflex increase in the activity of the neurohormonal parameters • fluid retention

Chapter **10**

Diabetic dyslipidaemia

10. Diabetic dyslipidaemia

- **the typical lipid profile abnormalities in diabetic patients are ↑ TG, ↑ VLDL-C, ↓ HDL-C, followed by ↑ TC and ↑ LDL-C**
- qualitative changes of lipoproteins including increased prevalence of small dense LDL-C particles with ↑ serum apo B concentration (Type B pattern) and enhanced atherogenicity
- associated factors such as hypertension, altered platelet function, oxidation and glycation of proteins and lipoproteins, hyperinsulinaemia, insulin resistance, altered immunological responses markedly enhance the risk of atherosclerosis in diabetic patients
- as in non-diabetic patients, other secondary causes of hyperlipidaemia such as hypothyroidism and the use of β-blockers and diuretics should be excluded

10.1 Hypercholesterolaemia

- TC reflects mainly endogenous cholesterol production, and fasting is not required for its determination; however, it may be influenced by acute illnesses (e.g. TC starts to fall 24 hours after myocardial infarction)
- TC mainly consists of HDL-C (protective) and LDL-C (atherogenic)
- HDL-C is measured and LDL-C is usually calculated from the Friedewald's equation:

$$[LDL\text{-}C] = [TC] - [HDL\text{-}C] - \{[TG]/2.2\}$$ in mmol/l if [TG] <4.5 mmol/l

- see 3.5.2 for target values

10.2 Hypertriglyceridaemia

- reflects exogenous fat consumption, hence fasting value is required
- related to hyperinsulinaemia, physical inactivity, poor glycaemic control and increased alcohol intake
- inversely proportional to HDL-C
- increased risk of pancreatitis if >10 mmol/l
- independent risk factor for coronary arterial disease if coexisting LDL-C/HDL-C ≥ 5

10.3 Treatment of hyperlipidaemia

- weight reduction if overweight
- regular exercise (2–3 times per week, lasting 20–60 minutes each time using major muscle groups)
- low fat diet
  - reduce dietary fat intake <20% of total caloric intake (saturated fat <10%)
  - reduce intake of animal fats, fatty cuts of meat (veal, beef, chicken skin), dairy products (butter, cheese, ice-cream), egg yolks, seafood (prawns, oysters, lobsters, crabs, squids), organ meats (brains, liver, heart), fast food (e.g. hamburgers, pizzas), coconut oil, egg noodles, baked food (e.g. cakes, cookies, biscuits)
  - reduce frequency of eating out
  - eat a balanced diet (see Chapter 5)
- the above aspects should be emphasized to patients to avoid unnecessary pharmacological intervention which may introduce an inappropriate sense of security and drug reliance in patients
- **an adequate period of at least 2–3 months of dietary treatment and 2 abnormal lipid levels are recommended before commencement of drugs**
- optimizing glycaemic control, increasing physical activity, stopping β blockers and diuretics, if appropriate, may improve hyperlipidaemia, especially ↑ TG

10.3.1 Predominant hypercholesterolaemia

- **a complete lipid profile (TC, HDL-C, TG) is required in the management of diabetic dyslipidaemia, especially if pharmacological intervention is considered** (see 3.4.2 for target values)
  - a) hydroxymethylglutaryl-coenzyme A (HMG-CoA) reductase inhibitor
    - up-regulate the LDL-C receptor with ↑ clearance of LDL-C and IDL-C (intermediate density lipoprotein cholesterol)
    - associated with regression of atheromatous plaque in coronary arteries and reduction of cardiovascular mortality and events
    - in the Scandinavian Simvastatin Survival Study (4S), treatment with simvastatin was associated

with 45% reduction in total mortality in diabetic patients with established coronary heart disease compared with placebo
- uncommon side effects include myalgia (with or without ↑ muscle enzymes, e.g. creatine phosphate kinase (CPK)) and abnormal liver function test
- ↑ risk of myositis if combined with gemfibrozil or nicotinic acid
- e.g. **lovastatin 10 mg o.d. to 40 mg b.d.**
   simvastatin 5–40 mg nocte
   pravastatin 10–40 mg o.d.
   atorvastatin 5–80 mg o.d.
   rosuvastatin 10–20 mg daily

b) bile acid sequestrant (resin)
- proven agent to reduce mortality from ischaemic heart disease in non-diabetic patients
- low toxicity due to non-absorbance but constipation and flatulence may reduce compliance
- may worsen hypertriglyceridaemia
- e.g **cholestyramine 4 g b.d.–8 g q.d.s.**

c) ezetimibe
- a cholesterol absorption inhibitor
- 10 mg once daily preparation
- reduces LDL-C, TC and TG, and increases HDL-C
- as monotherapy or in combination with statins or fibrates
- useful especially in homozygous familial hyper-lipidaemia in combination with high-dose statin to achieve LDL-C target

d) resistant cases of hypercholesterolaemia may improve with combination treatment of cholestyramine and HMG-CoA reductase inhibitors

10.3.2 Predominant hypertriglyeridaemia

- **respond favourably to weight reduction, exercise, improved glycaemic control and alcohol restriction**
   a) fibric acid derivatives
   - reduce hepatic synthesis of VLDL-C which is TG rich
   - may increase HDL-C
   - e.g. **gemfibrozil 600–1200 mg daily**
      fenofibrate 200–400 mg daily
      benzafibrate 200 mg t.d.s.–400 mg nocte

- b) nicotinic acid derivatives
    - ↓ lipolysis and the production of free fatty acid which is the precursor of VLDL-C
    - reduce LDL-C and TG and ↑ HDL-C but nicotinic acid may worsen glycaemic control and ↑ plasma urate level
    - e.g. **nicotinic acid 0.5–2 g t.d.s.**
        acipimox 250 mg t.d.s.
        (acipimox preferred)

10.3.3 Mixed dyslipidaemia (↑ TG and ↑ LDL-C)

- **HMG-CoA reductase inhibitors or fibrates depending on the predominant abnormality**
- combination treatment of fibrates (or nicotinic acid) and cholestyramine
- cautious use of HMG-CoA reductase inhibitors and fibrates in resistant cases

10.4 Summary of approaches to diabetic patient with dyslipidaemia

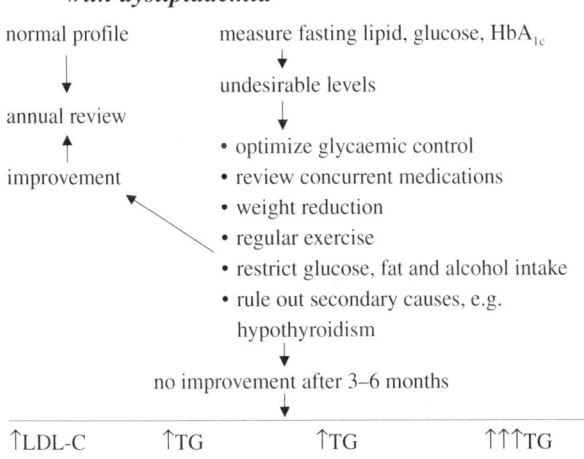

↑LDL-C	↑TG ↓HDL-C	↑TG ↓HDL-C ↑LDL-C	↑↑↑TG
• HMG-CoA reductase inhibitors • ezetimibe • resin	• fibrates • ezetimibe • acipimox	• fibrates • HMG-CoA reductase inhibitors • ezetimibe • acipimox • fibrates + resin	• fibrates • fat restriction (<10% of calories) • acipimox

- fish oils rich in the long-chain, highly polyunsaturated ω3 fatty acids may be tried if conventional treatment has failed or cannot be tolerated
- **patients with hyperlipidaemia requiring combination therapy should preferably be assessed and managed by specialists**

10.5 Treatment levels and cost-effectiveness of lipid lowering drugs

	Dietary treatment	Treatment level (LDL-C)	Target level (LDL-C)
USA National Cholesterol Education Programme (NCEP)			
established CHD or cardiovascular disease	6 weeks	≥3.4 mmol/l	<2.6 mmol/l
≥2 CVSRFs	3–6 months	≥4.1 mmol/l	<3.4 mmol/l
1 CVSRF	6–12 months	≥4.9 mmol/l	<4.1 mmol/l
British guidelines			
secondary prevention	6 weeks	≥3.4 mmol/l	<2.6 mmol/l
primary prevention	6–12 months	≥5.1 mmol/l (multiple risk factors) ≥6.1 mmol/l (no risk factor)	<4.1 mmol/l

CHD = coronary heart disease
CVSRF = cardiovascular risk factor

- interactions between plasma lipid levels and other cardiovascular risk factors are more important than absolute levels
- accepted risk factors for coronary heart disease (diabetes mellitus, hypertension or BP ≥140/90 mmHg, left ventricular hypertrophy, smoking, HDL-C <0.9 mmol/l, premature cardiovascular death in parents, siblings and offspring aged less than 60 years)
- HDL-C >1.4 mmol/l and a pre-menopausal state are protective factors against CHD
- lipid lowering drugs are most cost-effective in patients at

high risk for CHD taking into consideration the quality of life

- marked variability in terms of cost-effectiveness of HMG-CoA reductase inhibitors depending on patient characteristics
  - £136,000 in men aged 45–64 years with no history of CHD and a TC level >6.5 mmol/l treated for 10 years
  - on average, £32,000 in patients with pre-existing CHD and a TC level >5.4 mmol/l treated for 10 years
    - £6,000 in men aged 55–64 years who had a history of myocardial infarction with a TC level >7.2 mmol/l
    - £361,000 in women aged 45–54 years with angina and a TC level of 5.5–6.0 mmol/l
- optimization of other CVSRFs, e.g. control of BP, body weight and diabetes, cessation of smoking and use of β blockers and aspirin may be more cost-effective than use of lipid lowering drugs
- the aim of treatment with lipid lowering drugs is to complement and not to replace dietary treatment

Chapter ***11***

Peri-operative management

11. Peri-operative management

11.1 General principles

- pre-operatively
  - stabilize diabetes whenever possible before surgery, patients treated with oral agents may require stabilization with insulin
  - ensure availability of rapid and regular bedside measurement of BG using haemostix (H'stix) during surgery and peri-operatively
  - full physical examination with particular emphasis on the cardiovascular system to ensure fitness for operation
  - plan for early morning surgery
  - stop long acting sulphonylureas (e.g. chlorpropamide) and biguanides (metformin) for at least 24 to 48 hours before surgery
  - omit short acting oral agents on the morning of operation
- peri-operatively
  - for stable patients or patients treated with diet alone who undergo minor procedures, plain 0.9% normal saline (NS) or 5% dextrose (D_5) with H'stix monitoring during operation may suffice
  - for moderate or major operations, commence glucose-insulin-electrolyte infusion with frequent H'stix monitoring during operation, preferably hourly
  - give intravenous infusion of 0.5–1.5 u regular insulin per hour and 1.5–2 mg glucose/kg/min (approximately 5 g glucose in 100 ml 5% dextrose or 50 ml 10% dextrose hourly for a 50 kg man)
  - add electrolytes accordingly (daily requirement: 50–70 mmol/day of potassium; 100–150 mmol/day of sodium)
- post-operatively (when patient is kept nil by mouth)
  - regular subcutaneous insulin and H'stix 4–6 hourly, adjust dose according to H'stix reading
  - if BG remains persistently high ($\geq$14 mmol/l) and particularly in the presence of ketonuria, switch over to IV insulin administration using either a glucose-insulin-electrolytes regimen (see 11.2.2) or insulin pump (see 12.1.3) and adjust infusion rate of insulin and fluid accordingly

- post-operatively (patient eating)
    - for patients previously treated with oral agents, re-introduce oral drugs when dietary intake is satisfactory, may need to stabilize on insulin if major operation has been performed (e.g. regular insulin 4–6 hourly p.r.n. or b.d. intermediate acting insulin)
    - for insulin-treated patients, re-introduce insulin at ½ or ⅓ of the maintenance dose (preferably given as b.d. intermediate acting insulin) and gradually increase to full maintenance dosage
    - if glycaemic control is unsatisfactory on simple regimen, consider change to intensive therapy, e.g. regular insulin 15–30 minutes before each meal with intermediate/long acting insulin at bedtime
- **there is no standard protocol for peri-operative management of diabetes, frequent monitoring and consequent adjustment of insulin dosage and dextrose infusion are of paramount importance, monitor plasma electrolytes and measure laboratory plasma glucose values to correlate with H'stix regularly (preferably once daily)**
- in general, intravenous regular insulin is preferred if the patient is kept nil by mouth while subcutaneous regular insulin should be given 15–30 minutes before meal with or without long acting insulin to control basal glycaemia if the patient is eating

11.2 Type 2 diabetes — poorly controlled (must establish control before surgery)

11.2.1 Non-urgent surgery

a. diet ± oral drugs as outpatient
b. re-admit when control is satisfactory
c. then follow Type 2 diabetes — well controlled protocol

11.2.2 Moderately urgent surgery

a. diet ± b.d. intermediate acting insulin as in-patient
b. monitor H'stix q.i.d.
c. arrange operation when diabetes is under control — follow Type 2 diabetes — well controlled protocol

11.2.3   Urgent surgery

a.   IV insulin infusion using sliding scale — use DKI drip
     (11.3.2) or insulin pump (12.1.3)
b.   fluid and electrolyte (K^+) replacement
c.   monitor electrolytes and chart BG hourly
d.   do ***not*** operate until BG <16.7 mmol/l unless un-
     avoidable
e.   see also 11.4.1 (Type 1 diabetes — poorly controlled for
     emergency surgery)

11.3   Type 2 diabetes — well controlled

11.3.1   Minor surgery

a.   fast overnight
b.   operation preferably in the morning
c.   omit oral drugs on day of operation
d.   omit chlorpropamide or biguanide for at least 24 hours
     before operation
e.   pre-operatively, set up IV solution according to H'stix

H'stix (mmol/l)	Infusion
≤8.9	0.9% NaCl only
>8.9–11.1	regular insulin 5 u with 500 ml of D_5 Q6H (i.e. ~1 u/hr)
>11.1–16.7	regular insulin 8–10 u with 500 ml of D_5 Q6H (i.e. ~1.5 u/hr)
>16.7	regular insulin 12 u with 500 ml of D_5 Q6H and preferably delay operation (i.e. ~2 u/hr)

f.   monitor H'stix
     – with premedication
     – during operation
     – on return from theatre
     – Q4H thereafter
g.   post-operatively when diet is resumed, re-start oral drugs
     if H'stix is satisfactory or give regular insulin 15 to 30
     minutes before meal time, e.g. 5 u if H'stix >11.1–16.7
     mmol/l or 8–10 u if H'stix >16.7 mmol/l or change to b.d.
     intermediate acting insulin until BG stabilize

11.3.2 Major surgery (not eating ≥24 hours)

a. fast overnight
b. operation preferably in the morning
c. omit oral drugs on day of operation
d. omit chlorpropamide or biguanide for at least 24 hours before operations
e. IV infusion of 10% dextrose/potassium/insulin (DKI drip) to theatre

   e.g. 500 ml D_{10} Q6H IV infusion with

H'stix Q6H (mmol/l)	Regular insulin (u/500 ml)	K^+ (mmol/500 ml)
4.4–8.9	5 (~1 u/h)	5
>8.9–11.1	10 (~1.5 u/h)	10
>11.1–16.7	15 (~2 u/h)	15
>16.7–22.2	20 (~3 u/h)	20 and re-assess

   add 5–10 ml 23.4% NaCl (20–40 mmol Na^+) for every 500 ml D_{10}

f. check BG and plasma Na^+, K^+ post-operatively and adjust replacement of electrolytes accordingly
g. monitor H'stix Q6H and continue DKI drip
h. discontinue IV infusion and restart oral drugs if oral intake is satisfactory
i. insulin may be required temporarily during the post-operative stage, consider switching back to oral agents if total daily insulin requirement is less than 20 u

11.4 Type 1 diabetes — poorly controlled

11.4.1 For emergency surgery

NEVER operate until diabetes is at least partially controlled.

a. fast patient
b. IV saline/K^+ — rate of infusion determined by hydration state and plasma electrolytes
c. insulin pump — 6 u/hr IV initially
d. monitor and chart BG hourly
e. monitor K^+ hourly initially + ECG
f. keep insulin at 6 u/hr until BG <16.7 mmol/l and then adjust to maintain 5–10 mmol/l

g.   do not give dextrose until BG <16.7 mmol/l
h.   operate when general condition and BG are stable

If you operate on "acute abdomen" due to diabetes ketoacidosis, the mortality is extremely high!

11.5 Type 1 diabetes — well controlled

11.5.1 Minor surgery (eating evening meal)

a.   fast overnight
b.   operation preferably in the morning
c.   usual intermediate or long acting insulin evening before
d.   on day of operation, omit regular insulin in the morning
e.   monitor H'stix regularly, set infusion pre-operatively

H'stix (mmol/l)	Infusion
4.4–8.9	regular insulin 2–3 u in 500 ml D_5 Q6H (i.e. ~0.5 u/hr)
>8.9–11.1	regular insulin 5 u in 500 ml D_5 Q6H (i.e. ~1 u/hr)
>11.1–16.7	regular insulin 8–10 u in 500 ml D_5 Q6H (i.e. ~1.5 u/hr)
>16.7	regular insulin 12 u in 500 ml D_5 Q6H (i.e. ~2 u/hr) and delay operation until control is established

f.   post-operatively, monitor H'stix Q6H and continue IV fluid ± insulin
g.   decide evening insulin dosage depending upon progress
     e.g. ½ of usual p.m. intermediate acting insulin dosage depending on dietary intake, give additional regular insulin 30 minutes before meal if indicated

11.5.2 Major surgery (not eating >24 hours)

a.   fast overnight
b.   operation in the morning, omit insulin on day of operation
c.   DKI drip Q6H (see 11.3.2) or insulin infusion pump with sliding scale (see 12.1.3)
d.   monitor and chart BG hourly peri-operatively
e.   adjust infusion rate to maintain BG between 6.7 and 11.1 mmol/l

Chapter **12**

Diabetic emergencies

12. Diabetic emergencies

- **close monitoring and appropriate adjustment of insulin, fluid and electrolytes regimen are of paramount importance in the management of diabetic emergencies**

12.1 Diabetic ketoacidosis (DKA)

- usually in Type 1 diabetes but may occur in Type 2 diabetes especially in association with intercurrent illnesses
- diagnostic criteria for DKA:
  - plasma glucose >10 mmol/l
  - pH < 7.35
  - low $[HCO_3^-]$
  - high anion gap
  - positive serum or urine ketones
- see 12.1.7 for atypical DKA

12.1.1 Flow chart

- hourly vital signs including BP, pulse rate (PR), central venous pressure (CVP)
- hourly urine volume
- amounts/timing of insulin administration
- blood glucose (BG) and biochemistry (pH, Na^+, K^+, HCO_3^-, Cl^- to allow calculation of anion gap = $([Na^+] + [K^+]) - ([HCO_3^-] + [Cl^-])$ which should be less than 20 mmol/l. An anion gap ≥ 20 mmol/l suggests the presence of lactates, ketones, poisons (e.g. alcohol, glycerol, salicylates), sulphur-containing amino acids in rhadomyolysis or sulphates and phosphates in uraemia
- seek underlying causes including septic workup, CXR, ECG

12.1.2 Rehydration

- average fluid deficit 4–6 litres
- give 1–2 litres of 0.9% NaCl in first 2 hours (cautious use in patients with compromised cardiac status preferably with CVP monitoring)
- rate of additional fluid depend on urine output and clinical assessment of fluid state (e.g. BP, PR, CVP)

- if plasma Na^+ ≥150 mmol/l, change to 5% dextrose or 0.45% NaCl or 0.18% NaCl solution depending on severity of ↑Na^+
- change to D_5 when BG drops to 14 mmol/l or less
  a) as source of free water
  b) prophylaxis against development of cerebral oedema
  c) to allow continued infusion of sufficient insulin to normalize the anion gap and prevents further ketogenesis

12.1.3 Insulin (regular insulin)

- IV insulin infusion via pump + hourly H'stix (if possible, get plasma K^+ result before starting insulin)
- preparation of insulin pump with 50 ml total volume:
  a) • 48 ml of 0.9% NaCl
     • 0.5 ml U100 regular insulin (= 50 units)
     • 1.5 ml human albumin or patient's serum
                        or
  b) • 49.5 ml haemacel + 0.5 ml regular insulin (50 units)
  – final insulin concentration in syringe = 1 unit/ml
  – insulin pump scale

H'stix (mmol/l)	Regular insulin (u/hr)
4.4–6.7	0.5
>6.7–8.9	1
>8.9–11.1	2
>11.1–16.7	3
>16.7–27.8	4
>27.8	6 or more if necessary

  – adjust infusion scale according to response of H'stix monitoring, maintain H'stix between 6–11 mmol/l
- start with 0.1 u/kg/hr or 6 u/hr, increase if BG does not fall after 2 hours
- when BG ↓ to <28 mmol/l, adjust insulin dosage according to H'stix result and maintain H'stix value between 6–11 mmol/l (2–3 u/hr is usually needed)
- **avoid complete cessation of insulin infusion, there may be rapid decompensation resulting in DKA due**

to a lack of suppression of lipolysis by insulin especially in unstable Type 1 diabetic patients

- change to subcutaneous insulin when the patient is fully conscious and eats well, overlap administration of subcutaneous insulin with insulin pump for 2 hours or so to allow the former to take effect
- if the patient is insulin resistant, e.g. requiring ≥10 u/hr to control glycaemia, consider:
  - venous access (the drip may be out!)
  - pump failure or expired insulin
  - uncontrolled or occult sepsis
  - other known insulin resistant states, e.g. acromegaly, Cushing's syndrome, etc.
- **persistent ketonuria or failure to correct acidosis despite improvement of BG suggests inadequate insulin action to inhibit lipolysis. Increased amount of insulin with additional glucose infusion will be necessary rather than replacement with HCO_3^- only**
- the anion gap, which must be monitored throughout the course of DKA, should narrow with treatment although ketonuria may persist as the patient improves due to increased formation of acetone which is a ketone body but not an acid

12.1.4 Bicarbonate (HCO_3^-)

- HCO_3^- should *not* be given unless pH <7.1 for the following reasons:
  a) precipitate rapid intracellular K^+ shift with hypokalaemia
  b) tissue anoxia due to a shift of O_2 dissociation curve
  c) cerebral acidosis due to ↓ pH in the cerebrospinal fluid
  d) sodium overload
- for pH <7.1, give 50–100 mmol $NaHCO_3$ with 15–30 mmol K^+ slowly (e.g. over 2 hours) (omit K^+ if plasma K^+ ≥4.5 mmol/l)
- repeat pH 30 minutes after the HCO_3^- infusion
- 1 ml 8.4% $NaHCO_3$ = 1 mmol HCO_3^-
- give 1.4% $NaHCO_3$ if hyperosmolar (e.g. plasma Na^+ ≥ 150 mmol/l), prepare by adding 50 ml 8.4% $NaHCO_3$ in 250 ml of D_5 if 1.4% solution is not available

- **persistent acidosis may indicate inadequate insulin dosage or other causes of metabolic acidosis**
- avoid using large amount of $NaHCO_3^-$ (>100 mmol/l) especially in hypertonic form

12.1.5 Electrolyte replacement

- **obtain plasma K^+ result (which may be normal, $\uparrow$ or $\downarrow$) as soon as possible to guide further management, in any case, plasma K^+ result should be made available within 1–2 hours of starting insulin treatment, ECG may be useful in assessing severity of hyperkalaemia (T waves changes)**
- preferably give 0.9% NaCl only until K^+ is known
- **monitor electrolytes 1–2 hourly initially for 4–6 hours then every 2–4 hours until stable**
- **both insulin treatment and reversal of acidosis can cause marked intracellular shift of K^+ leading to potentially fatal hypokalaemia, early K^+ replacement is usually required once insulin treatment is commenced**
- adjust plasma K^+ replacement according to renal function
- change to dextrose solution when BG is less than 14 mmol/l to provide carbohydrate substrate and prevent development of hyperchloraemic acidosis due to excessive use of NaCl solution
- change to hypotonic saline if plasma Na^+ continues to increase, earlier change to glucose infusion may be necessary in hypernatraemic state (plasma $Na^+ \geq 150$ mmol/l)
- severe hypernatraemia or electrolyte abnormalities may lead to rhabdomyolysis with marked $\uparrow$ CPK and renal impairment

12.1.6 Ancillary treatment and follow up

- PO_4 replacement — optional, replacement not proven of clinical value
- nasogastric tube for unconscious patient to prevent aspiration especially if paralytic ileus or gastric dilatation are also present
- catheterization may be required to monitor urine output

- close monitoring of fluid status using PR/BP, consider insertion of CVP line especially in elderly patients to facilitate fluid replacement
- hourly H'stix and 4 hourly plasma electrolytes during the first 24 hours and until stable — more frequent if necessary
- look for underlying causes including sepsis, tuberculosis, and secondary causes of diabetes
- beware of dramatic reductions of insulin requirement once acute episode of DKA settles, honeymoon period with minimal or no insulin requirement may ensue later
- **close monitoring of the clinical status of the patient with appropriate management of fluid, electrolytes and insulin are mandatory. Hyperglycaemia is only one target of the management, electrolytes and the acid base balance are equally if not more important**
- remember to identify and manage underlying causes if relevant

12.1.7 Atypical DKA

- euglycaemic DKA
  - may occur if good hydration is maintained or when insulin is given but the dosage is inadequate for a ketogenic stress
  - usually occurs in patients who are young, well hydrated, treated with insulin, during intercurrent illness or in pregnancy
  - correct diagnosis is important, treatment is similar to those for DKA
- non-ketotic DKA
  - there are 3 ketone bodies: β-hydroxybutyrate, acetoacetate and acetone
  - DKA with elevated anion gap but predominant β-hydroxybutyrate formation, which is not measured in the urine test for ketones (nitroprusside reaction)
  - usually occurs in situations of tissue hypoxaemia, e.g. sepsis, hypotension or shock; or in alcoholic
  - should evaluate for concomitant lactic acidosis
- alkalaemic DKA
  - in severe vomiting, diuretic use or alkali ingestion

- mixed pattern of metabolic alkalosis and metabolic acidosis
- clue is marked elevation of anion gap and a pH that is higher than expected for the size of anion gap

12.2 Hyperosmolar non-ketotic coma (HNKC)

- occurs more frequently in the elderly with neglected Type 2 diabetes and develops over more prolonged periods
- associated with severe dehydration, and may be precipitated by the use of diuretics, cerebrovascular accidents, myocardial infarction or renal disease
- hyperglycaemia with absent or minimal ketones formation and acidosis
- plasma osmolality > 330 mOsmol/l (normal: 280–295). Osmolality can be measured or calculated [2 ($Na^+ + K^+$) + BG + urea in mmol/l]

12.2.1 Rehydration

- 6–10 litres of fluid commonly required. Watch plasma Na^+ very carefully: if plasma $Na^+ \geq 150$ mmol/l, start with 0.45% NaCl solution. **Great care is needed to avoid hypernatraemia during treatment**

12.2.2 Insulin pump

- **BG can ↓ significantly just with adequate rehydration**
- patients are usually more sensitive to insulin treatment
- insulin dosage on sliding scale, ↓ by half of that for DKA (see 12.1.3)
- avoid rapid normalization of BG in the first 24 hours to ↓ risk of cerebral oedema

12.2.3 Other treatments

- similar to those for DKA

12.3 Lactic acidosis

- metabolic acidosis (pH ≤ 7.25) with absent or minimal ketones formation, increased anion gap ≥ 20 mmol/l (see

12.1.1.) due to an increased concentration of circulating lactate > 5 mmol/l (normal fasting value: 0.5–1.3 mmol/l)

- a condition with high mortality especially if accompanied by circulatory collapse and respiratory failure
- fatigue of respiratory muscle may ensue rapidly requiring mechanical ventilation
- lactate is an end product of incomplete oxidation which is normally converted to glucose and HCO_3^- by oxidation in the mitochondria within the liver and kidney
- lactic acidosis occurs due to an imbalance between the production and removal of lactate
- causes of lactic acidosis:

  Type A:
  - increased anaerobic glycolysis as a result of tissue anoxia or hypotension (e.g. cardiac failure, sepsis, cyanide, nitroprusside, carbon monoxide poisoning)

  Type B:
  - impaired mitochondrial function due to biguanides
  - reduced capacity of liver or kidney to remove lactate
  - may also occur in cases of uncontrolled diabetes, alcoholism, parenteral nutrition with large amounts of fructose, neoplasia and toxins (e.g. salicylates, methanol, ethylene glycol, epinephrine)

- **correction of hypoxia, haemodynamic abnormalities and treatment of underlying cause (e.g. sepsis) are fundamental**:
  - maintain adequate airway and good oxygenation (may need mechanical ventilation)
  - fluid treatment to restore tissue perfusion
  - antibiotic coverage if indicated

- large amount of alkali ($NaHCO_3$) may be required to maintain the plasma HCO_3^- at 8–10 mmol/l and pH above 7.1 although this is not always associated with clinical benefits. Current evidence is against the routine use of IV $NaHCO_3$ which significantly increases $PaCO_2$ and reduces plasma ionized calcium level

- diuretics or dialysis with a HCO_3^- buffered fluid may be required to prevent circulatory overload, hyperosmolality and hypernatraemia

- avoid over-correction of acidosis (aim at $HCO_3^- \approx 15$

mmol/l) due to potential overshoot of pH with recovery of lactate metabolism and HCO_3^- production
- dichloroacetate may be useful but information is still limited
- **in most cases of metformin-related lactic acidosis, contraindications to its use (renal, hepatic, cardiac or respiratory dysfunction or alcoholism) have been present**
- phenformin is associated with high risk of lactic acidosis but is still available in China and some underdeveloped countries

Chapter **13**

Gestational diabetes mellitus

13. Gestational diabetes mellitus (GDM)

- pregnancy is associated with a decrease in maternal insulin sensitivity
- the human placental lactogen, progesterone, prolactin and cortisol have been shown to reduce the peripheral actions of insulin, hence, the maintenance of glucose tolerance in pregnancy requires a 2- to 3-fold increase in post-prandial maternal insulin secretion
- fasting plasma glucose concentration falls throughout pregnancy because of increasing placental uptake of glucose and reduced hepatic glucose output while post-prandial values rise due to impaired glucose disposal

13.1 Definition and prevalence

- GDM is defined as glucose intolerance of variable severity with onset or first recognition during pregnancy irrespective of whether or not insulin is used for treatment or the condition persists after pregnancy
- the possibility that glucose intolerance may have antedated the pregnancy is not considered as an exclusion criterion for this definition
- the prevalence of GDM is 2–3% and varies markedly amongst different studies, depending on diagnostic criteria and ethnic groups
- Asians appear to have a higher prevalence of about 8%, and it was about 5.8% in the Prince of Wales Hospital in 1996

13.2 Screening and diagnosis

- the lack of consensus on the diagnostic criteria for GDM makes it difficult to compare study results from different countries

13.2.1 Screening

- American Diabetes Association (ADA) recommends that all pregnant women should be screened for glucose intolerance with special attention to those with increased risk:
  - overweight
  - over 30 years of age
  - family history of DM (first-degree relatives)

- past obstetric history of unexplained stillbirth or macrosomic babies (>4 kg)
- glycosuria
- screening test (ADA recommendation 1996): 50 g of oral glucose given without regard to time of the last meal or time of day. Venous plasma glucose 1 hour later ≥7.8 mmol/l requires full diagnostic OGTT
- if low risk and asymptomatic, perform screening test between 24th and 28th weeks of gestation
- if high risk, screen early or perform full diagnostic test

13.2.2 Diagnostic OGTT

- some centres omit screening test due to low sensitivity and perform OGTT if clinically indicated
- no current concensus on diagnostic criteria, variable in glucose load, number of blood samplings and plasma glucose cut-off values
- options of diagnostic OGTT:
  - O'Sullivan and Mahan criteria — 100 g oral glucose load, 2 or more out of the 4 venous plasma glucose values met or exceeded: fasting plasma glucose (FPG) 5.8 mmol/l; 1-hr 10.6 mmol/l; 2-hr 9.2 mmol/l; 3-hr 8.1 mmol/l
  - Royal Australian College of O&G — 75g oral glucose load, diagnostic if FPG >5.5 mmol/l and/or 2-hr PG ≥8.0 mmol/l
  - Japan Society of O&G — 75 g oral glucose load, 2 or more of the venous PG values exceeded: FPG 5.6 mmol/l; 1-hr 10.0 mmol/l; 2-hr 8.3 mmol/l
  - WHO (IGT or DM) — as in non-pregnant population
- the Australian criteria have been used at the Prince of Wales Hospital's Obstetrics and Gynaecology Department since 1996

13.3 Obstetric and perinatal implications

- increased risk of fetal and neonatal complications including macrosomia, birth trauma, neonatal hypoglycaemia and intra-uterine death
- poor glycaemic control in the first weeks of pregnancy especially in those with pre-existing diabetes is

associated with increased risks of congenital malformation of infants and spontaneous abortion

- the incidence of major congenital anomalies, e.g. caudal regression, spina bifida, situs inversus, ureter duplex, in infants of diabetic mothers is 3–6 times more common than infants of non-diabetic mothers
- increased perinatal mortality rate in GDM is still controversial
- increased maternal risks of operative intervention, infection and polyhydramnios

13.4 Management

- good diabetic control is necessary before pregnancy, during pregnancy and labour to minimize maternal, fetal and neonatal complications
- some Type 2 diabetic patients may need insulin treatment for optimal glycaemic control before conception
- strict peri-conceptional diabetic control is essential to minimize congenital fetal malformation or spontaneous abortion
- **close surveillance of mother and fetus is most important**
- with optimal care, the maternal and fetal outcome should be as normal as that in non-diabetic population

13.4.1 Maternal management

- monitoring of urinary glucose is not useful due to reduced renal threshold for glucose excretion in pregnancy leading to glucosuria despite euglycaemia
- **self-monitoring of capillary blood glucose is mandatory**
- dietary therapy remains the cornerstone of diabetic treatment
- proper nutritional counselling by dietitians, education by diabetes nurses including techniques of self blood glucose monitoring and self injection of insulin are necessary
- aim to maintain FPG ≤5.5 mmol/l and 2-hr post-prandial PG ≤7.0 mmol/l
- dietary treatment should include the provision of adequate calories and nutrients to meet the needs of pregnancy

- intake of sucrose and other caloric sweeteners should be limited; non-caloric sweeteners may be used in moderation
- insulin is needed if target glycaemic control is not achieved with dietary therapy
- oral hypoglycaemic agents are not accepted during pregnancy due to risks of fetal hyperinsulinaemia and neonatal hypo-glycaemia from placental transfer

13.4.2 Fetal management

- regular fetal surveillance includes ultrasound assessment of dates and fetal morphology, monitoring for macrosomia, polyhydramnios and antepartum cardiotocography
- monitoring can be performed on an outpatient basis, hospital admissions are required if maternal or fetal complications develop
- unless maternal or fetal complications arise, delivery should be delayed till 38 weeks of gestation or later in order to reduce complications from pre-term delivery. Spontaneous labour is preferred to avoid failed induction but some patients may need induction of labour earlier because of development of complications, e.g. preeclampsia, polyhydramnios. They need thorough assessment by obstetricians and diabetologists for fetal well being and maternal glycaemic status
- aims to deliver fetus vaginally, Caesarean section is reserved for obstetric indications or fetal macrosomia
- for spontaneous vaginal delivery, frequent intrapartum monitoring of maternal glycaemic status, continuous fetal heart rate monitoring and uterine contraction assessment should be performed. Intravenous DKI infusion is required for Caesarean section

13.4.3 Neonatal management

- early notification of the neonatologist (and paediatric surgeon for surgically correctable fetal abnormalities) prior to delivery
- infants of diabetic mothers have an increased risk of respiratory distress syndrome
- neonatal hypoglycaemia is common in the first 48 hours

after delivery, the infant may be lethargic and have dyspnoea or seizure
- frequent monitoring of neonatal glycaemic status to detect hypoglycaemia is essential and early feeding is encouraged
- watch out for other neonatal problems include hypocalcaemia, hypomagnesaemia, poor feeding, hyperbilirubinaemia, polycythaemia
- breast-feeding should be encouraged except in Type 2 diabetic patients on oral hypoglycaemic agents

13.4.4 Postpartum management

a) Short-term:
- pre-existing diabetes: resume pre-pregnant diabetic treatment
- GDM: stop all antenatal diabetic treatment and monitor glycaemic status to ensure normoglycaemia before discharge
- postnatal education on contraception and family planning, low dose combined oral contraceptive pills (OCP) may be prescribed but close surveillance of glycaemic control is required
- the progestogen component of the OCP may induce insulin resistance while the oestrogen component may increase blood pressure and thrombogenic tendency in predisposed individuals, there are very few long-term studies on the use of these agents in Asian Type 2 diabetic women or those with a history of GDM
- short-term studies in non-Caucasian women including Chinese show increased incidence of glucose intolerance in women with a history of GDM who received low dose OCP compared to women with no such history

b) Long-term:
- women with a history of GDM have a 50% chance of having GDM again in subsequent pregnancies
- in one study, 17 years after the initial diagnosis of GDM, 40% of women became diabetic compared with 10% in an age-matched control group who had normal glucose tolerance in pregnancy, risk factors include:
  – increased body weight
  – increased age

- higher parity
- more severe degrees of and/or early onset of glucose intolerance during pregnancy
- GDM in 2 or more pregnancies
- women in whom GDM is diagnosed should be followed in the postpartum period to detect diabetes early in its course:
  - measures glycaemic status at 6 weeks postpartum using the ADA or WHO criteria (see Chapter 2)
  - regular follow-up 1–2 yearly with blood glucose testing
  - early antenatal booking and careful assessment in next pregnancy with early OGTT
  - maintain ideal body weight, weight reduction if already overweight
  - avoid smoking
- infants of diabetic mothers are also at increased risk of developing childhood obesity and diabetes or GDM in the future

Chapter **14**

Prevention of diabetes mellitus

14. Prevention of diabetes mellitus

- diabetes mellitus is a major public health problem causing significant morbidity and mortality with far-reaching socio-economical implications
- **over half of diabetic subjects remain undiagnosed and many are receiving suboptimal or unsupervised treatment**
- it has been predicted that the number of diabetic subjects in Asia will exceed 250 million by the year 2000, of whom 100 million will be in mainland China

14.1 Primary prevention

- aims at preventing the onset of diabetes mellitus
- achieved mainly by public health education to the whole population or selected groups on the nature of diabetes mellitus and its impact on health
  - health education should begin in school to encourage a healthy lifestyle
- lifestyle modification to improve insulin resistance (see also Chapter 5):
  - correction and prevention of obesity
  - avoidance of a high-fat diet
  - advocate intake of diet with a high carbohydrate content from unrefined sources and a high intake of soluble fibre
  - avoidance or cautious use of diabetogenic drugs, e.g. β-blockers, diuretics, steroids and oral contraceptive pills, especially in subjects at risk of developing diabetes
  - increased physical activity

14.2 Secondary prevention

- aims at identifying undiagnosed cases to allow early intervention
- screening of high risk groups by primary health care providers:
  - strong family history of Type 2 diabetes
  - history of gestational diabetes mellitus
  - history of large-for-dates babies
  - history of impaired glucose tolerance

    – change from traditional (rural or active) to westernized
      (urbanized or sedentary) lifestyles
    – features of the "Metabolic Syndrome" — hyperten-
      sion, hyperlipidaemia especially hypertriglyceri-
      daemia and obesity, especially central

14.3 Tertiary prevention

- aims at preventing the onset or minimizing the progression of diabetic complications
- integrated system involving different levels of diabetes
  care including:
  - family doctors
  - hospital diabetologists
  - diabetes educators (nurse specialists, dietitians,
    podiatrists, community nurses)
  - other specialists such as ophthalmologists, orthopaedic
    surgeons, nephrologists
  - social workers and community support group
  - paramedical health care professionals (physio-
    therapists and occupational therapists)

14.4 Multidisciplinary care in diabetes mellitus

- self-care
  - modify lifestyle
  - maintain normal body weight
  - perform self blood or urine glucose monitoring
  - attend regular medical follow-up
  - learn about diabetes and adopt a positive attitude
- primary health care providers
  - provide and reinforce diabetes education
  - assist patients in their self-care
  - adjust medical therapy
  - regularly make assessment for complications, car-
    diovascular risk factors and metabolic control
  - identify problems that require hospital attention
- hospital diabetes centre or clinic
  - assist primary health care providers in the provision of
    diabetes care, especially at or close to diagnosis and at
    times when changes in therapy are required to optimize
    glycaemic control

- complement diabetes care in the community by providing comprehensive diabetes assessment and therapeutic patient education
- establish lines of communication with primary health care providers
- update knowledge of other health care providers in diabetes
- provide expertise for diagnosis and management of diabetic complications
- provide emergency care during periods of crisis
- provide ancillary care services, e.g. dietitians, podiatrists
- provide monitoring and quality assurance programmes for diabetes care within the community
- assist in the planning of strategies for diabetes care
- continue to research into the pathogenesis of the disease, develop and evaluate new treatment and method of care delivery

Appendix I

Body mass index (BMI) chart

Body Mass Index (kg/m²)   **MALE**

Weight (Kg)	Height (cm)										Weight (Lbs)
	145	150	155	160	165	170	175	180	185	190	
50	24	22	21	20	18	17	16	15	15	14	110
52	25	23	22	20	19	18	17	16	15	14	114
54	26	24	22	21	20	19	18	17	16	15	119
56	27	25	23	22	21	19	18	17	16	16	123
58	28	26	24	23	21	20	19	18	17	16	128
60	29	27	25	23	22	21	20	19	18	17	132
62	29	28	26	24	23	21	20	19	18	17	136
64	30	28	27	25	24	22	21	20	19	18	141
66	31	29	27	26	24	23	22	20	19	18	145
68	32	30	28	27	25	24	22	21	20	19	150
70	33	31	29	27	26	24	23	22	20	19	154
72	34	32	30	28	26	25	24	22	21	20	159
74	35	33	31	29	27	26	24	23	22	20	163
76	36	34	32	30	28	26	25	23	22	21	167
78	37	35	32	30	29	27	25	24	23	22	172
80	38	36	33	31	29	28	26	25	23	22	176
82	39	36	34	32	30	28	27	25	24	23	180
84	40	37	35	33	31	29	27	26	25	23	185
86	41	38	36	34	32	30	28	27	25	24	189
88	42	39	37	34	32	30	29	27	26	24	194
90	43	40	37	35	33	31	29	28	26	25	198
Weight (Kg)	4'9"	4'11"	5'1"	5'3"	5'5"	5'7"	5'9"	5'11"	6'1"	6'3"	Weight (Lbs)
	Height (ft/in)										

Ideal body weight < 25 Kg/m²   Borderline 25-27 Kg/m²   Obese ≥ 27 Kg/m²

Body Mass Index (kg/m²)   **FEMALE**

Weight (Kg)	Height (cm)										Weight (Lbs)
	145	150	155	160	165	170	175	180	185	190	
50	24	22	21	20	18	17	16	15	15	14	110
52	25	23	22	20	19	18	17	16	15	14	114
54	26	24	22	21	20	19	18	17	16	15	119
56	27	25	23	22	21	19	18	17	16	16	123
58	28	26	24	23	21	20	19	18	17	16	128
60	29	27	25	23	22	21	20	19	18	17	132
62	29	28	26	24	23	21	20	19	18	17	136
64	30	28	27	25	24	22	21	20	19	18	141
66	31	29	27	26	24	23	22	20	19	18	145
68	32	30	28	27	25	24	22	21	20	19	150
70	33	31	29	27	26	24	23	22	20	19	154
72	34	32	30	28	26	25	24	22	21	20	159
74	35	33	31	29	27	26	24	23	22	20	163
76	36	34	32	30	28	26	25	23	22	21	167
78	37	35	32	30	29	27	25	24	23	22	172
80	38	36	33	31	29	28	26	25	23	22	176
82	39	36	34	32	30	28	27	25	24	23	180
84	40	37	35	33	31	29	27	26	25	23	185
86	41	38	36	34	32	30	28	27	25	24	189
88	42	39	37	34	32	30	29	27	26	24	194
90	43	40	37	35	33	31	29	28	26	25	198
Weight (Kg)	4'9"	4'11"	5'1"	5'3"	5'5"	5'7"	5'9"	5'11"	6'1"	6'3"	Weight (Lbs)
	Height (ft/in)										

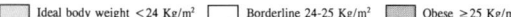

Ideal body weight < 24 Kg/m²   Borderline 24-25 Kg/m²   Obese ≥ 25 Kg/m²

Appendix **II**

Carbohydrate exchange list

To enable patients to have a regular intake of carbohydrate in the diet, an exchange system is used. Portions of foods listed below all contain the same amount of carbohydrate (10 grams = 40 kcal). Each 10 grams of carbohydrate is called an EXCHANGE.

Food	Handy measure	Weight
Dairy products		
milk, whole or skim	1 glass	240 ml
milk powder, whole	4 level tablespoons	25 g
skim	4 level tablespoons	20 g
evaporated milk, unsweetened	6 tablespoons	90 ml
yoghurt, natural	1 small carton	160 ml
Bread		
wholemeal	1/2 slice	20 g
white	1/2 slice	20 g
Life Bread (Garden)	1 slice without crust	20 g
Grains and flours		
rice, cooked	1 round tablespoon	30 g
vermicelli, cooked	1/4 medium bowl	35 g
noodle, cooked	1/4 medium bowl	50 g
spaghetti, cooked	1/3 medium bowl	30 g
macaroni, cooked	1/3 medium bowl	55 g
chapatti, wholemeal	1 small plate size	20 g
flour, wholemeal	2 level tablespoons	15 g
flour, white	1½ level tablespoons	15 g
Cereals		
oatmeal, raw	2 level tablespoons	15 g
all bran	3 level tablespoons	15 g
Weetabix	1 piece	15 g
shredded wheat	1 tablespoon	10 g
muesli (unsweetened)	2 level tablespoons	15 g
cornflakes	1/2 medium bowl	12 g
Rice Krispies	1/2 medium bowl	12 g
Biscuits		
large digestive	1 piece	15 g
crispbread	2 pieces	15 g
oatcake	1 round piece	15 g
plain or semi-sweet	2 pieces	15 g

Chinese dim sums

plain *cheung fun*	1 roll	50 g
beef *cheung fun*	1 roll	30 g
BBQ pork bun	1/2 bun	80 g
siu mai	4 pieces	60 g
shrimp dumpling	4 pieces	80 g
taro dumpling, fried	1½ pieces	40 g
spring roll	3/4 roll	30 g
chicken and curdsheet roll	2 pieces	100 g

*   1 tablespoon is a 15 ml spoon. 1 teaspoon is a 5 ml spoon.

** patients will be given a meal plan incorporating the amount and distribution of carbohydrate throughout the day

References

Alberti KGMM, Zimmet PZ, for the WHO Consultation. Definition, diagnosis and classification of diabetes mellitus and its complications. Part 1: Diagnosis and classification of diabetes mellitus provisional report of a WHO consultation. *Diabetic Medicine* 1998;15:539–53.

ALLHAT Officers and Coordinators for the ALLHAT Collaborative Research Group. The Antihypertensive and Lipid-Lowering Treatment to Prevent Heart Attack Trial. Major outcomes in high-risk hypertensive patients randomized to angiotensin-converting enzyme inhibitor or calcium channel blocker vs diuretic: The Antihypertensive and Lipid-Lowering Treatment to Prevent Heart Attack Trial (ALLHAT). *Journal of American Medical Association* 2002;288:2981–97.

ALLHAT Officers and Coordinators for the ALLHAT Collaborative Research Group. The Antihypertensive and Lipid-Lowering Treatment to Prevent Heart Attack Trial. Major outcomes in moderately hypercholesterolemic, hypertensive patients randomized to pravastatin vs usual care: The Antihypertensive and Lipid-Lowering Treatment to Prevent Heart Attack Trial (ALLHAT-LLT). *Journal of American Medical Association* 2002;288:2998–3007.

American Diabetes Association. Standards of medical care for patients with diabetes mellitus. *Diabetes Care* 1998;21 (suppl. 1):S23–S31.

American Diabetes Association. Standards of medical care for patients with diabetes mellitus. *Diabetes Care* 2004; 27:S15–S35.

Anderson PJ, Chan JCN, Chan YL, Tomlinson B, Young RP, Lee Z, et al. Visceral fat and cardiovascular risk factors in Chinese NIDDM patients. *Diabetes Care* 1997;20:1854–8.

Assal J-Ph. Educating the diabetic patient: difficulties encountered by patients and health care providers who have to teach NIDDM and IDDM patients. *Concepts for the ideal diabetes clinic*. Berlin, New York: W. de Gruyter, 1992: 73–87.

Ballantyne CM, Houri J, Notarbartolo A, Melani L, Lipka LJ, Suresh R, Sun S, LeBeaut AP, Sager PT, Veltri EP; Ezetimibe Study Group. Effect of ezetimibe coadministered with atorvastatin in 628 patients with primary hyper-cholesterolemia: a prospective, randomized, double-blind trial. *Circulation* 2003;107:2409–15.

Björntorp P. Metabolic implications of body fat distribution. *Diabetes Care* 1991;14:1132–43.

Bolli GB, Owens DR. Insulin glargine. *Lancet* 2000;356:443–5.

Brenner BM, Cooper ME, de Zeeuw D, Keane WF, Mitch WE, Parving H-H, Remuzzi G, Snapinn SM, Zhang Z, Shahinfar S, for the RENAAL Study Investigators. Effects of losartan on renal and cardiovascular outcomes in patients with type 2 diabetes and nephropathy. *New England Journal of Medicine* 2001;345:861–9.

Chan JC, Cheung JC, Stehouwer CD, Emeis JJ, Tong PC, Ko GT, Yudkin JS. The central roles of obesity-associated dyslipidaemia, endothelial activation and cytokines in the Metabolic Syndrome — an analysis by structural equation modelling. *International Journal Obesity Related Metabolic Disorders* 2002;26:994–1008.

Chan JC, Ng MC, Critchley JA, Lee SC, Cockram CS. Diabetes mellitus — a special medical challenge from a Chinese perspective. *Diabetes Research and Clinical Practice* 2001;54 (Suppl 1):S19–S27.

Chan JCN, Chan KW, Ho LLT, Fuh MMC, Lee CH, Sheaves R, et al. An Asian multi-centre clinical trial to assess the efficacy and tolerability of acarbose compared with placebo in Type 2 diabetic patients previously treated with diet. *Diabetes Care* 1998;21:1058–61.

Chan JCN, Chan NN, Cockram CS. Diabetes Mellitus. *Principles and Practice of Clinical Medicine in Asia*, ed. J. Sung, et al. Hong Kong: Lippincott Williams & Wilkins 2002, p429–62.

Chan JCN, Cheung CK, Cheung MYF, Swaminathan R, Critchley JAJH, Cockram CS. Abnormal albuminuria as a predictor of mortality and renal impairment in Chinese patients with NIDDM. *Diabetes Care* 1995;18:1013–4.

Chan JCN, Cheung CK, Cockram CS, Critchley JAJH, Swaminathan R, Nicholls MG. Atrial natriuretic peptide (ANP) and renin-angiotensin-aldosterone system in patients with non-insulin-dependent diabetes (NIDDM). *Journal of Human Hypertension* 1994;8:451–6.

Chan JCN, Cheung CK, Swaminathan R, Nicholls MG, Cockram CS. Obesity, abnormal albuminuria and hypertension among Hong Kong Chinese with non-insulin-

dependent diabetes. *Postgraduate Medical Journal* 1993;
69:204–10.

Chan JCN, Cheung JCK, Lau EMC, Woo J, Chan AYW, Swaminathan R, et al. The Metabolic Syndrome in Hong Kong Chinese — the interrelationships among its components analyzed by structural equation modeling. *Diabetes Care* 1996;19:953–9.

Chan JCN, Chow CC, eds. *Living positively with diabetes* (in Chinese, 2nd edition). Hong Kong: The Chinese University Press, 1996.

Chan JCN, Cockram CS. Diabetes in the Chinese population and its implications for health care. *Diabetes Care* 1997; 20:1785–90.

Chan JCN, Cockram CS, Critchley JAJH. Drug-induced disorders of glucose metabolism — mechanisms and management. *Drug Safety* 1996;15:135–56.

Chan JCN, Cockram CS, Nicholls, MG, Cheung CK, Swaminathan R. Comparison of enalapril and nifedipine in treating non-insulin-dependent diabetes associated with hypertension: one year analysis. *British Medical Journal* 1992;305:981–5.

Chan JCN, Critchley JAJH, Cockram CS. Patients with diabetes mellitus. Management of hypertension. *Medical Progress* 1997;April:19–26.

Chan JCN, Critchley JAJH, Ho CS, Nicholls MG, Cockram CS, Swaminathan R. Atrial natriuretic peptide (ANP) and urinary dopamine output in non-insulin-dependent diabetes mellitus. *Clinical Science* 1992;83:247–53.

Chan JCN, Critchley JAJH, Tomlinson B, Chan TYK, Cockram CS. Antihypertensive and anti-albuminuric effects of losartan potassium and felodipine-ER in Chinese elderly hypertensive patients with or without NIDDM. *American Journal of Nephrology* 1997;17:72–80.

Chan JCN, Lau M, Wong RYM, Chow CC, Yeung VTF, Loo KM, et al. Delivery of diabetes care — the experience at the Prince of Wales Hospital. *Hospital Authority Quality Bulletin* 1997;2:3–21.

Chan JCN, Tomlinson B, Critchley JAJH, Cockram CS, Walden RJ. Metabolic and hemodynamic effects of metformin and glibenclamide in normotensive NIDDM patients. *Diabetes Care* 1993;16(7):1035–8.

Chan JCN, Wong RYM, Cheung CK, Lam P, Chow CC, Yeung

VTF, et al. Accuracy, precision and user-acceptability of self blood glucose monitoring machines. *Diabetes Research and Clinical Practice* 1997;36:91–104.

Chan JCN, Yeung VTF, Cheung CK, Swaminathan R, Cockram CS. The inter-relationships between albuminuria, plasma albumin concentration and indices of glycaemic control in non-insulin-dependent diabetes mellitus. *Clinica Chimica Acta* 1992;210:179–85.

Chan JCN, Yeung VTF, Chow CC, Cockram CS. Diabetes mellitus — epidemiology and pathogenesis. *Hong Kong Practitioner* 1996;18:270–80.

Chan JCN, Yeung VTF, Chow CC, Cockram CS. Diagnosis and management of diabetes mellitus. *Hong Kong Practitioner* 1996;18:331–45.

Chan JCN, Yeung VTF, Chow CC, Cockram CS. Treatment of diabetic complications and associated conditions. *Hong Kong Practitioner* 1996;18:379–90.

Chan JCN, Yeung VTF, Chow CC, Ko GTC, Mackay IR, Rowley MJ, et al. Pancreatic β cell function and antibodies to glutamic acid decarboxylase (anti-GAD) in Chinese patients with insulin-dependent diabetes mellitus (IDDM). *Diabetes Research and Clinical Practice* 1996;32:27–34.

Chan JCN, Yeung VTF, Leung DHY, Tomlinson B, Nicholls MG, Cockram CS. The effects of enalapril and nifedipine on carbohydrate and lipid metabolism in NIDDM. *Diabetes Care* 1994;17:859–62.

Chan NN, Brain HPS, Feher MD. Metformin-associated lactic acidosis: a rare or very rare clinical entity? *Diabetic Medicine* 1999;16(4):273–81.

Chan NN, Fauvel NJ, Feher MD. NSAID and metformin: a cause for concern? *Lancet* 1998;352:201.

Chan NN, Feher MD. Long-term ACE inhibitor therapy in diabetic nephropathy: potential hazard? *Diabetic Medicine* 1998;5:524.

Chan NN, Feher MD. Metformin and peri-operative risk. *British Journal of Anaesthesia* 1999;83:540–1.

Chan NN, Feher MD. Metformin and the ageing diabetic patients. *Age and Ageing* 2000;29:187.

Chan NN, Hurel SJ. Potential impact of a new non-invasive glucose monitor: the Glucowatch Biographer. *Practical Diabetes International* 2002;19:97–100.

Chan NN, Tong PC, So WY, Leung WY, Chiu CK, Chan JC.

The metabolic effects of insulin and rosiglitazone combination therapy in Chinese type 2 diabetic patients with nephropathy. *Medical Science Monitor* 2004;10:PI44–8.

Chan WK, Chan TYK, Luk WK, Leung VKS, Li TH, Critchley JAJH. A high incidence of cough in Chinese subjects treated with angiotensin converting enzyme inhibitors. *European Journal of Clinical Pharmacology* 1993;44:299–300.

Chiasson JL, Josse RG, Gomis R, Hanefeld M, Karasik A, Laakso M; STOP-NIDDM Trial Research Group. Acarbose treatment and the risk of cardiovascular disease and hypertension in patients with impaired glucose tolerance: the STOP-NIDDM trial. *Journal of American Medical Association* 2003;290:486–94.

Chobanian AV, Bakris GL, Black HR, Cushman WC, Green LA, Izzo JL Jr, Jones DW, Materson BJ, Oparil S, Wright JT Jr, Roccella EJ; National Heart, Lung, and Blood Institute Joint National Committee on Prevention, Detection, Evaluation, and Treatment of High Blood Pressure; National High Blood Pressure Education Program Coordinating Committee. The Seventh Report of the Joint National Committee on Prevention, Detection, Evaluation, and Treatment of High Blood Pressure: the JNC 7 report. *Journal of American Medical Association* 2003; 289:2560–72.

Chow CC, Sorensen JP, Tsang LWW, Cockram CS. Comparison of insulin with or without continuation of oral hypoglycaemic agents in the treatment of secondary failure in NIDDM patients. *Diabetes Care* 1995;18:307–14.

Cockram CS, Lau JTF, Chan AYW, Woo J, Swaminathan R. Assessment of glucose tolerance test criteria for diagnosis of diabetes in Chinese subjects. *Diabetes Care* 1992;15:988–90.

Cockram CS, Woo J, Lau E, Chan JCN, Chan AYW, Lau J, et al. The prevalence of diabetes mellitus and impaired glucose tolerance among Hong Kong Chinese adults of working age. *Diabetes Research and Clinical Practice* 1993;21:67–73.

Collins R, Armitage J, Parish S, Sleight P, Peto R; Heart Protection Study Collaborative Group. Effects of cholesterol-lowering with simvastatin on stroke and other major vascular events in 20536 people with cerebrovascular disease or other high-risk conditions. *Lancet* 2004;363:757–67.

Dahlof B, Devereux RB, Kjeldsen SE, Julius S, Beevers G,

de Faire U, Fyhrquist F, Ibsen H, Kristiansson K, Lederballe-Pedersen O, Lindholm LH, Nieminen MS, Omvik P, Oparil S, Wedel H, for the LIFE study group. *Lancet* 2002;359:995–1003.

DeFronzo RA, Ferranninni E. Insulin resistance: a multifaceted syndrome responsible for NIDDM, obesity, hypertension, dyslipidemia and atherosclerotic cardiovascular disease. *Diabetes Care* 1991;14:173–94.

Diabetes Control and Complications Trial Research Group, The. The effect of intensive treatment of diabetes on the development and progression of long-term complications in insulin-dependent diabetes mellitus. *New England Journal of Medicine* 1993;329:977–86.

Ewing DJ, Clarke BF. Diagnosis and management of diabetic autonomic neuropathy. *British Medical Journal* 1982;285: 916–8.

Expert Committee on the Diagnosis and Classification of Diabetes Mellitus, The. Report of the Expert Committee on the Diagnosis and Classification of Diabetes Mellitus. *Diabetes Care* 1997;20:1183–97.

Galloway JA. Treatment of NIDDM with insulin agonists or substitutes. *Diabetes Care* 1990;13:120–39.

Gerich JE. Novel insulins: expanding options in diabetes management. *American Journal of Medicine* 2002;113: 308–16.

Heart Outcome Prevention Evaluation (HOPE) Study Investigators. Effects of rampril on cardiovascular and microvascular outcomes in people with diabetes mellitus: results of the HOPE study and MICRO-HOPE substudy. *Lancet* 2000;355:253–9.

Hoffman L. Gestational diabetes mellitus. *Medical Journal of Australia* 1998;168:140.

James WP, Astrup A, Finer N, Hilsted J, Kopelman P, Rossner S, Saris WH, Van Gaal LF. Effect of sibutramine on weight maintenance after weight loss: a randomised trial. STORM Study Group. Sibutramine Trial of Obesity Reduction and Maintenance. *Lancet* 2000;356:2119–25.

Ko BCB, Lam KSL, Wat NMS, Chung SSM. An (A-C)n dinucleotide repeat polymorphic marker at the 5' end of the aldose reductase gene is associated with early-onset diabetic retinopathy in NIDDM patients. *Diabetes* 1995; 44:727–32.

Ko GT, Chan JC, Cockram CS. Change of glycaemic status in Chinese subjects with impaired fasting glycaemia. *Diabetic Medicine* 2001;18:745–8.

Ko GT, Cockram CS, Critchley JA, Chan JC. Glycaemic control and obesity are the major determinants of diabetic dyslipidaemia in Hong Kong Chinese. *Diabetes and Metabolism* 2001;27:637–44.

Ko GTC, Chan JCN, Lau E, Woo J, Cockram CS. Fasting plasma glucose as a screening test for diabetes and its relationship with cardiovascular risk factors in Hong Kong Chinese. *Diabetes Care* 1997;20:170–2.

Ko GTC, Chan JCN, Woo J, Lau E, Yeung VTF, Chow CC, et al. Glycosylated hemoglobin and cardiovascular risk factors in Chinese with normal glucose tolerance. *Diabetic Medicine* 1998;15:513–8.

Ko GTC, Chan JCN, Woo J, Lau E, Yeung VTF, Chow CC, et al. The reproducibility of oral glucose tolerance test in Chinese. *Annals of Clinical Biochemistry* 1998;35:62–7.

Ko GTC, Chan JCN, Woo J, Lau E, Yeung VTF, Chow CC, et al. Simple anthropometric indexes and cardiovascular risk factors in Chinese. *International Journal of Obesity and Related Metabolic Disorders* 1997;21:995–1001.

Ko GTC, Chan JCN, Woo J, Lau EMC, Yeung VTF, Chow CC, et al. The effect of age on cardiovascular risk factors in Chinese women. *International Journal of Cardiology* 1997;61:221–7.

Ko GTC, Chan JCN, Yeung VTF, Chow CC, Li JKY, Lau MSW, et al. Antibodies to glutamic acid decarboxylase in young Chinese diabetic patients. *Annals of Clinical Biochemistry* 1998;35:761–7.

Ko GTC, Chan JCN, Yeung VTF, Chow CC, Tsang LWW, Li JKY, et al. Combined use of a fasting plasma glucose concentration and HbA_{1c} or fructosamine predicts the likelihood of having diabetes in high risk subjects. *Diabetes Care* 1998;21:1221–5.

Ko GTC, Chow CC, Li CY, Yeung VTF, Cockram CS. Insulin-dependent diabetes mellitus presenting as diabetic ketoacidosis in pregnancy. *The Australian and New Zealand Journal of Obstetrics and Gynaecology* 1995; 35:321–2.

Ko GTC, Yeung VTF, Chan JCN, Chow CC, Li JKY, So WY, et al. Plasma fibrinogen concentration in a Chinese population. *Atherosclerosis* 1997;131:211–7.

Kohner EM, Porta M. Introduction to the protocols on screening and treatment of diabetic retinopathy. *European Journal of Ophthalmology* 1991;1:46–54.

Kreisberg RA. Pathogenesis and management of lactic acidosis. *Annual Review of Medicine* 1984;35:181–93.

Lam KSL, Tiu SC, Tsang MW, Ip TP, Tam SCF. Acarbose in NIDDM patients with poor control on conventional oral agents. *Diabetes Care* 1998;21:1154–8.

Lee SC, Ko GT, Li JK, Chow CC, Yeung VT, Critchley JA, Cockram CS, Chan JC. Factors predicting the age when type 2 diabetes is diagnosed in Hong Kong Chinese subjects. *Diabetes Care* 2001;24:646–9.

Leung WY, Neil Thomas G, Chan JC, Tomlinson B. Weight management and current options in pharmacotherapy: orlistat and sibutramine. *Clinical Therapeutics* 2003;25(1): 58–80.

Lewis EJ, Hunsicker LG, Bain RP, Rhode RD, for the Collaborative Study Group. The effect of angiotensin converting enzyme inhibition on diabetic nephropathy. *New England Journal of Medicine* 1993;329:1456–62.

Linn T, Bretzel RG. Diabetes in pregnancy. *European Journal of Obstetrics & Gynecology and Reproductive Biology* 1997;75:37–41.

Lithell HOL. Effect of antihypertensive drugs on insulin, glucose and lipid metabolism. *Diabetes Care* 1991;40: 203–9.

Liu KH, Chan YL, Chan WB, Kong WL, Kong MO, Chan JC. Sonographic measurement of mesenteric fat thickness is a good correlate with cardiovascular risk factors: comparison with subcutaneous and preperitoneal fat thickness, magnetic resonance imaging and anthropometric indexes. *International Journal of Obesity Related Metabolic Disorders* 2003;27:1267–73.

Martin FIR. The diagnosis of gestational diabetes. *Medical Journal of Australia* 1991;155:112.

Mogensen C. Microalbuminuria predicts clinical proteinuria and early mortality in maturity onset diabetes. *New England Journal of Medicine* 1984;310:356–60.

Mogensen CE, Keane WF, Bennet PH, Jerums G, Parving HH, Passa P, et al. Prevention of diabetic renal disease with special reference to microalbuminuria. *Lancet* 1995;346: 1080–4.

Nutrition recommendations and principles for people with diabetes mellitus. *Journal of the American Dietetic Association* 1994;94:504–6.

Ohkubo Y, Kishikawa H, Araki E, Miyata T, Isami S, Motoyoshi S, et al. Intensive insulin therapy prevents the progression of diabetic microvascular complications in Japanese patients with NIDDM: a randomised prospective 6-year study. *Diabetes Research and Clinical Practice* 1995;28:103–17.

Parving H-H, Lehnert H, Brochner-Mortensen J, Gomis R, Andersen S, Arner P, for the Irbesartan in Patients with Type 2 Diabetes and Microalbuminuria Study Group. The effect of irbesartan on the development of diabetic nephropathy in patients with type 2 diabetes. *New England Journal of Medicine* 2001;345:870–8.

Pasui K, McFarland KF. Management of diabetes in pregnancy. *American Family Physician* 1997;55:2731–8, 2742–4.

Pfeifer MA, Beach DE, Schrage J, Gelber D, Miller-Crain G, Kuperstein Chasen J, et al. Treatment and practical management of diabetic somatic neuropathy: a working philosophy for the forgotten complication of diabetes. *International Diabetes Monitor* 1993;5:1–7.

Pinhas-Hamiel O, Dolan LM, Zeitler PS. Diabetic ketoacidosis among obese African-American adolescents with NIDDM. *Diabetes Care* 1997;20:484–6.

Piwernetz K, Home PD, Snorgaard O, Antsiferov M, Staehr-Johansen K, Krans M. For the DiabCare Monitoring Group of the St. Vincent Declaration Steering Committee. Monitoring the targets of the St. Vincent declaration and the implementation of quality management in diabetes care: the DiabCare initiative. *Diabetic Medicine* 1993;10:371–7.

Prisant LM. Clinical trials and lipid guidelines for type II diabetes. *Journal of Clinical Pharmacology* 2004;44:423–30.

Pugh HA, Wagner ML, Sawyer J, Ramirez G, Tuley M, Friedberg SJ. Is combination sulfonylurea and insulin therapy useful in NIDDM patients? A metaanalysis. *Diabetes Care* 1992;15:953–9.

Pyörälä K, Pedersen TR, Kjekshus J, Faergeman O, Olsson AG, Thorgeirsson G, The Scandinavian Simvastatin

Survival Study (4S) Group. Cholesterol lowering with simvastatin improves prognosis of diabetic patients with coronary heart disease: a subgroup analysis of the Scandinavian Simvastatin Survival Study (4S). *Diabetes Care* 1997;20: 614–20.

Ravid M, Lang R, Rachmani R, Lishner M. Long-term renoprotective effect of angiotensin-converting enzyme inhibition in non-insulin-dependent diabetes mellitus. A 7-year follow-up study. *Archives of Internal Medicine* 1996; 156:286–9.

Ravid M, Neumann L, Lishner N. Plasma lipids and the progression of nephropathy in diabetes mellitus type II: effect of ACE inhibitors. *American Journal of Kidney Diseases* 1995;47:907–10.

Ravid M, Savin H, Jutrin I, Bental T, Katz B, Lishner M. Long-term stabilizing effect of angiotensin-converting enzyme inhibition on plasma creatinine and on proteinuria in normotensive type II diabetic patients. *Annals of Internal Medicine* 1993;118:577–81.

Rossetti L, Giaccari A, DeFronzo RA. Glucose toxicity. *Diabetes Care* 1990;13:610–30.

Rowe DJF, Dawnay A, Watts GF. Microalbuminuria in diabetes mellitus: review and recommendations for the measurement of albumin in urine. *Annals of Clinical Biochemistry* 1990;27:297–312.

Smith PR, Dronsfield MJ, Mijovic CH, Hattersley AT, Yeung VTF, Cockram CS, et al. The mitochondrial tRNA[Leu(UUR)] A to G 3243 mutation is associated with insulin-dependent and non-insulin-dependent diabetes in a Chinese population. *Diabetic Medicine* 1997;14:1026–31.

Snow V, Aronson MD, Hornbake ER, Mottur-Pilson C, Weiss KB; Clinical Efficacy Assessment Subcommittee of the American College of Physicians. Lipid control in the management of type 2 diabetes mellitus: a clinical practice guideline from the American College of Physicians. *Annals Internernal Medicine* 2004;140:644–9.

So WY, Tong PC, Ko GT, Leung WY, Chow CC, Yeung VT, Chan WB, Critchley JA, Cockram CS, Chan JC. Effects of protocol-driven care versus usual outpatient clinic care on survival rates in patients with type 2 diabetes. *American Journal of Managed Care* 2003;9:606–15.

Soedamah-Muthu SS, Colhoun HM, Abrahamian H, Chan NN,

Mangili R, Reboldi GP, Fuller JH; EURODIAB Prospective Complications Study Group. Trends in hypertension management in Type 1 diabetes across Europe, 1989/90–1997/99. *Diabetologia* 2002;45:1362–71.

SOLVD Investigators, The. Effect of enalapril on mortality and the development of heart failure in asymptomatic patients with reduced left ventricular ejection fractions. *New England Journal of Medicine* 1992;327:685–91.

Tatti P, Pahor M, Byington RP, Di Mauro P, Guarisco R, Strollo G, et al. Outcome results of the fosinopril versus amlodipine cardiovascular events randomized trial (FACET) in patients with hypertension and NIDDM. *Diabetes Care* 1998;21:597–603.

Tinker LF, Heins JM, Holler HJ. Commentary and translation: 1994 nutrition recommendations for diabetes. *Journal of the American Dietetic Association* 1994;94:507–11.

Tong PC, Lee KF, So WY, Ng MH, Chan WB, Lo MK, Chan NN, Chan JC. White blood cell count is associated with macro- and microvascular complications in Chinese patients with type 2 diabetes. *Diabetes Care* 2004;27:216–22.

Tong PC, Lee ZS, Sea MM, Chow CC, Ko GT, Chan WB, So WY, Ma RC, Ozaki R, Woo J, Cockram CS, Chan JC. The effect of orlistat-induced weight loss, without concomitant hypocaloric diet, on cardiovascular risk factors and insulin sensitivity in young obese Chinese subjects with or without type 2 diabetes. *Archive of Internal Medicine* 2002;162: 2428–35.

Torgerson JS, Hauptman J, Boldrin MN, Sjostrom L. XENical in the prevention of diabetes in obese subjects (XENDOS) study: a randomized study of orlistat as an adjunct to lifestyle changes for the prevention of type 2 diabetes in obese patients. *Diabetes Care* 2004;27:155–61.

Velussi M, Brocco E, Frigato F, Zolli M, Muollo B, Maioli M, et al. Effects of cilazapril and amlodipine on kidney function in hypertensive NIDDM patients. *Diabetes* 1996; 45:216–22.

Viberti G, Wheeldon NM; for the MicroAlbuminuria reduction With VALsartan (MARVAL) Study Investigators. Microalbuminuria Reduction with valsartan in patients with type 2 diabetes mellitus. *Circulation* 2002;106:672–8.

Wang Y, Ng MC, Lee SC, So WY, Tong PC, Cockram CS, Critchley JA, Chan JC. Phenotypic heterogeneity and associations of two aldose reductase gene polymorphisms with nephropathy and retinopathy in type 2 diabetes. *Diabetes Care* 2003;26:2410–5.

Williams B. Insulin resistance: the shape of things to come. *Lancet* 1994;344:521–4.

Woo J, Swaminathan R, Cockram C, Pang CP, Mak YT, Au SY, et al. The prevalence of diabetes mellitus and an assessment of methods of detection among a community of elderly Chinese in Hong Kong. *Diabetologia* 1987;30: 863–8.

Zimmet PZ. Challenges in diabetes epidemiology — from West to the rest. *Diabetes Care* 1992;15:232–52.